THE CREATION DIET

GOD'S PATTERN FOR HEALTH, HAPPINESS, AND HOLINESS

JOY CLARY BROWN

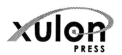

xulon PRESS

Dedication

I dedicate this book to:

God, the Creator of this beautiful world and the *author and finisher of our faith;*
I thank You for the inspiration that led to the writing of <u>The Creation Diet</u> and for the wonderful things You taught me during its progression.

My precious family;
To my husband, Wayne, and our children Meri Beth and her husband Thomas Howard, and Molly and her husband Christman Howard, I want to thank you for your constant encouragement that cheered me on to the finish. I offer a special "thank you" to Wayne and Molly for sacrificing your time and talents during many hours of tedious proofreading. The five of you help me experience life, love, and laughter daily.

To my deceased father, James Clary, who developed in me a hunger for God's Word and a thirst to know more I am grateful forever. Even in death he taught me the true meaning of life.
To my mother, Jeri Clary, I want to say you are the world's best cook! Thank you for all I've learned from you and for teaching me to eat and enjoy a variety of foods.
To my sister, Lynn, thank you for being a living example that nothing is impossible. I have marveled through the years as I watched you accomplish things to which you committed from teaching yourself to knit to becoming an accomplished harpist.
To my brother-in-law, Dr. Ron Sisk, your years of wonderful

chiropractic care have blessed me immeasurably. I owe my first exposure to natural health care to you and Lynn.

Judy Hughey Owens and the late Kay Freeman, and Rita Clary Harmon;
I could never express how God has used your friendships to bless and enrich my life since our teenage years. You have been the "bestest buddies" a girl could ever have.

Rita Stephan;
Thank you, Rita, for believing in The Creation Diet and for praying for it faithfully until its completion. You are a dear friend.

Don and Martha Hasty;
Thank you for helping the dream of this book become a reality. I pray that all your dreams come true as well.

Judy Rosenberg;
Thank you for mentoring me in the Jewish roots of Christianity. I owe much of the wisdom in this book to you. Thank you for all the books you loaned me as I was writing.

Jackie Owens, Rita Phillips, Loreni Cooper, Barbara Benton, Teresa Green, Kathy Blanton, David and Mildred Wellons and Sylvia Shirley
Thank you for your help and encouragement with this project through the years.

Vicki Wood;
Thank you for being my prayer partner and for telling me of Xulon Press. (Thank you, too, Dee Dee Wall.)

Women by Design;
Marie, Edna, Cherie, Tricia, Kimberly thank you for your encouragement and excitement over this project.

Marcia Parker;
Thank you for your assistance with the formatting of the chap-

ters. Your suggestions made the book more reader-friendly.

The late Sue Larzalere Williams;
   To Sue's family I want to say that your Nanna helped establish the first test group. I forever will be grateful to her for that and I miss her.

All the participants of the test groups;
   Thank you for your feedback that helped more than you probably realize. Your improved health convinced me that the principles of The Creation Diet needed to be shared with the world.

To all who will read The Creation Diet;
   May your lives be as enriched by reading this book as mine has been by writing it.

Special thanks to:
Iyse Lee, Author Support Manager, Xulon Press, for your help.

Pam Blume, Fair Forest Design, Boone, North Carolina, for the graphics.

Karen Ginn, Adjunct Instructor of English, Appalachian State University, Boone, North Carolina, for your help with proofing the manuscript.

Anita Laymon, In Laymon's Terms, Boone, North Carolina, for word processing support.

Dr. Jeff Clary, Spartanburg, South Carolina, for suggesting various resources to help with the medical research.

Dale Marie Shelton, Dale-Marie, A Portrait Studio, Boone, North Carolina, for the back cover photo.

Florence Littauer and Marita Littauer, Classervices, Albuquerque, New Mexico, for all you have taught me about writing and speaking.

Dr. William and Mary Mitchell, North Greenville College, Tigerville, South Carolina, for launching this ministry of writing and speaking.

Table of Contents

PREFACE

Diets and "miracle cures" abound in today's society. It seems that every few months "the answer" to ill health and/or obesity is lauded through the media. Bookstores and libraries devote large sections to "Diet/Nutrition" and "Health/Fitness," yet the resources often contradict each other concerning what is truly the answer to health and wholeness in life.

Modern lifestyles wreak devastation on the spiritual, mental/emotional, and physical well being of children, youth, and adults. The National Center for Health Statistics reports that 70% of all deaths in the United States are the result of heart disease or cancer, and 80% of those deaths are the direct result of lifestyle choices

As books and other health-related resources proliferate, diseases escalate at alarming rates. Multi-million dollar book sales verify that people are purchasing this genre of literature. However, national and international health seems to decrease as book sales increase. Could it be that conflicting messages about diet/nutrition/fitness could be part of the problem rather than the solution? How can a person discern the truth amidst the confusion?

Many wonderful biblically based health resources are available. However, even they can promote programs and principles that often contradict each other. Some are based on research of what people ate in biblical days. Others have been developed through observing the lifestyles of contemporary people, from varying countries and cultures, who are considered healthy. Still others take secular plans and support the principles with scripture.

How and where does a person find the plan that promotes ultimate health and well being in every area of life—spirit, soul, and body?

And God said. . .

Amazingly, God reveals this plan through the order in which He created the world. God's Word brought into existence the world and everything in it.

And God said. . .

Through the opening verses of the Bible He reveals, in sequential order of importance, the elements that will create—or re-create—health and wholeness in each of His creations. This revelation is simple, yet profound.

And God said. . . in the creation narrative how to live full and abundant lives—spirit, soul, and body.

The Creation Diet takes the order of the creation week and correlates each day's creations with health and wholeness spiritually (spirit), mentally/emotionally (soul) and physically (body). Each chapter presents a Biblical Application, a Nutritional Application, and a Spiritual Application and reveals choices that rob us of the benefits of God's creations. Each chapter, excluding the final chapter, concludes with seven devotionals associated with the creations addressed in the relative chapter.

The Creation Diet was tested in two groups of people of various ages, weights, and health conditions. The results were remarkable. Those who needed to lose weight lost significant amounts while others needing improvement in health conditions experienced results that astounded some in the medical community.

For example, one female participant lost 90 pounds in eight months and was taken off the anti-depression medicine she had been on for seven years. Several participants lost in excess of 50 pounds over a period of four months. The following excerpts are taken from testimonials supplied by members of the groups:

What a wonderful book that clearly shows God's plan for healthy eating! Thank you for sharing with us God's creation story for healthy living.

Angela Perry, Employee Health Nurse
Grand Strand Regional Medical Center

My name is Kent and I am a 48 year old male who in the last 15 years was diagnosed with Muscular Dystrophy. Since then, I have had one health problem after another—from three heart attacks to having full-blown Diabetes, taking five shots of insulin a day. Last summer I was told (after being rushed to the hospital and put on oxygen) that I was in my last days, and that I could die in a matter of days, weeks or months.

Of course, after hearing all of that, I gave up. But, thank God, Joy Clary Brown did not. It was not just her praying, because I know she does that without ceasing, but she asked me to try The Creation Diet. I argued with her that it would not make a differ-ence, but she kept after me. Thank God I did try it. . . I am now feel-ing the best that I have felt in years. I no longer have to take pills and insulin for the sugar. In fact, my sugar levels have so regulated that they are in the best control they have been for many years.

The most exciting part is not just that my lungs have changed or that my muscles have regained strength, it is also the fact that through the way I am eating—the fresh and steamed veggies, small amounts of fruit, less meat and the refined sugar gone—and so much more, the diet has changed my life and God has truly glori-fied His Word through the scripture. My wife and I thank Joy for allowing God to use her and work through her. My life is a true testimony of His glory and the gift of His diet.

Kent Hamilton, Speech Clinician

My name is Debi and I am Kent's wife. He and I owe so much to the Lord through His work in Joy Clary Brown and The Creation Diet. It has made a difference in our lives and I believe God and His direction through this diet actually saved Kent's life.

My testimony is the fact that I have lost over a hundred pounds. This has been the first eating plan in my life that did not feel like a diet, but a way of life… This new way of life eating has made the true taste of natural fruits and vegetables so good that the less I eat of processed sugars, the better I feel.

Being a woman, it seemed that my emotions were always running high. I experience the most benefit from The Creation Diet in that area. The closer I stay to the diet plan, the more even keeled I feel emotionally—and the energy is always there. I know God has blessed this work and I believe it can make a difference regardless of what your life is about. I thank Joy Clary Brown, and I thank my heavenly Father!

Debi Hamilton, Educator

We have three children: 16, 14 and 11 years old. Since we all have a tendency to be overweight, I was thrilled when asked to join The Creation Diet *test group. The only obstacle at the time was how I would get my children to eat vegetables the way they should... We began to change our habits, and the first week it was difficult, but when they felt good and had more energy, they were more enthused about it.*

We went on vacation and ate out everyday. When we came home we got back into our old habits. About two weeks later, all three of my children came to me at different times throughout the week complaining about how they felt and asked to start eating the way we were on The Creation Diet. *They said that while eating according to that plan they felt better, had more energy, and were all losing weight without even trying. God brings all things together!*

Susan Moore, Manager, *Little Body Builders*

I am flabbergasted that God's plan of creation shows, by its order, what our bodies need. How many times have we read those Bible verses but missed so much of their importance? Modern science now confirms the same order. That re-emphasized to me the relevance of God's Word to our present lives, and gives me a renewed appreciation of God's awesome, majestic power, plan and control over the most detailed parts of our beings.

What a revelation to recognize how many instances of foreshadowing of Jesus are presented in the Old Testament! These revelations from the author are God-given, eye openers to us in directing our actions in making ourselves more physically healthful and spiritually (faith) strengthened.

Verification from the Bible that this is the true way to handle nutrition is certainly the best motivation for putting this diet into practice.

Gladys Long, Retired Real Estate Broker

Joy Clary Brown's book, <u>The Creation Diet</u>, uncovered so many profound truths for me. I was amazed to see how, from the very beginning, God had a plan even about the best way for us to eat. If you never knew that God created the universe with you in mind, you will after you read this book.

Rita Gray Williams, Special Education Teacher

As with any health program, you should consult a health care professional before beginning <u>The Creation Diet</u>. My sincere desire is that <u>The Creation Diet</u> will bless the lives of those who read it as much as writing it has blessed and enriched my life. I am praying that God will make His plan known to you individually as you read <u>The Creation Diet</u>. My prayer will be also that you not only *read* about God's loving plan, but that you personally *experience* it! God loves you so much that even before He created you He provided the plan that would bless you with abundant life—spirit, soul, and body!

IN THE BEGINNING . . .

BIBLICAL APPLICATION

(Genesis 1:1-31-Genesis 2:3)

Genesis 1:1-31

1 In the beginning God created the heavens and the earth. 2 Now the earth was formless and empty, darkness was over the surface of the deep, and the Spirit of God was hovering over the waters. 3 And God said, "Let there be light," and there was light.

4 God saw that the light was good, and he separated the light from the darkness.

5 God called the light "day," and the darkness he called "night." And there was evening, and there was morning—the first day [original Hebrew—day one].

6 And God said, "Let there be an expanse between the waters to separate water from water." 7 So God made the expanse and separated the water under the expanse from the water above it. And it was so. 8 God called the expanse "sky." And there was evening, and there was morning—the second day.

9 And God said, "Let the water under the sky be gathered to one place, and let dry ground appear." And it was so. 10 God called the dry ground "land," and the gathered waters he called "seas." And God saw that it was good.

11 Then God said, "Let the land produce vegetation: seed bearing plants and trees on the land that bear fruit with seed in it, according to their various kinds." And it was so. 12 The land produced vegetation: plants bearing seed according to their kinds and trees bearing fruit with seed in it according to their kinds. And God saw that it was good. 13 And there was evening, and there was morning—the third day.

14 And God said, "Let there be lights in the expanse of the sky to separate the day from the night, and let them serve as signs to mark seasons and days and years, 15 and let them be lights in the expanse of the sky to give light on the earth." And it was so.

16 God made two great lights—the greater light to govern the day and the lesser light to govern the night. He also made the stars. 17 God set them in the expanse of the sky to give light on the earth, 18 to govern the day and the night, and to separate light from darkness. And God saw that it was good. 19 And there was evening, and there was morning—the fourth day.

20 And God said, "Let water teem with living creatures, and let birds fly above the earth across the expanse of the sky." 21 So God created the great creatures of the sea and every living and moving thing with which the water teems, according to their kinds, and every winged bird according to its kind. And God saw that it was good. 22 God blessed them and said, "Be fruitful and increase in number and fill the water in the seas, and let the birds increase on the earth." 23 And there was evening, and there was morning—the fifth day.

24 And God said, "Let the land produce living creatures according to their kinds: livestock, creatures that move along the ground, and wild animals, each according to its kind." And it was so. 25 God made the wild animals according to their kinds, the livestock according to their kinds, and all creatures that move along the ground according to their kinds. And God saw that it was good.

26 Then God said, "Let us make man in our image, in our likeness, and let them rule over the fish of the sea and the birds of the air, over the livestock, over all the earth, and over all the creatures that move along the ground."

27 So God created man in his own image, in the image of God he created him; male and female he created them. 28 God blessed them and said to them, "Be fruitful and increase in number; fill the earth and subdue it. Rule over the fish of the sea and the birds of the air and all the creatures that move on the ground."

29 Then God said, "I give you every seed-bearing plant on the face of the whole earth and every tree that has fruit with seed in it. They will be yours for food. 30 And to all the beasts of the earth and all the birds of the air and all the creatures that move on the ground—*everything that has the breath of life in it—I give every green plant for food." And it was so.*

31 God saw all that he had made, and it was very good. And there was evening, and there was morning—the sixth day.

Genesis 2:1-3

1 Thus the heavens and the earth were completed in all their vast array. 2 By the seventh day God had finished the work he had been doing; so on the seventh day he rested from all his work. 3 And God blessed the seventh day and made it holy, because on it he rested from all the work of creating that he had done.

Prologue

In the beginning. . . (Genesis 1:1), a fascinating phrase begins the incomparable Book that has guided millions of people through thousands of years.

In the beginning God. . . (Genesis 1:1), a concept that is affirmed throughout the Bible.

In the beginning God created the heavens and the earth. . . (Genesis 1:1), a truth that assures us of a definite, purposeful beginning to the world in which we live.

I invite you to join me in a fascinating journey that reveals step-by-step a beautiful path leading to total health and well being. Tucked away in the creation narrative is a powerful message showing how the order of God's creation of the world directly relates to our lives today. Through it we find the secret to health and wholeness.

May God bless you as you embark on one of the most exciting ventures of your life—The Creation Diet. *In the beginning,* and all chapters in between, I pray sincerely that this book will bring health and happiness to you, and honor to the One for whom and by whom you were created!

BALANCE AND PURPOSE

A basic order of balance can be seen in every aspect of life. God has ordained it so and has taken great care to cause it to happen. Even the smallest of details is arranged with balance and purpose in mind. For example, did you know that God designed the following:

An even number of rows on an ear of corn?
An even number of segments in an orange?
An even number of stripes on a watermelon rind?
An even number of grains on a wheat stalk?

Isn't that amazing?

Also, did you realize that no matter what the weather, the waves of the sea roll onto shore twenty-six times per minute? Sir Isaac Newton's third law of motion states that each action has an equal and opposite reaction. Even this basic theory of dynamics is further proof that balance is ordained by God and has a purpose. God never does anything by chance. He does everything with balance and purpose.

Isn't That Amazing?

One day, while mopping the kitchen floor, I had a revelation that led to the writing of this book. (I jokingly told my husband that perhaps there is something to the old adage, "Cleanliness is next to godliness.") I had become an avid student of nutrition. Specifically, the relationship between nutrition and the dietary laws in Genesis 1:29, Leviticus 11:9-12, Deuteronomy 14:3-8, and Deuteronomy 14:19 interested me. I realized there was a God-given correlation between those passages and modern nutritional research.

On that memorable day, I was amazed again by God's accuracy as I re-discovered the importance of word order in the Bible. Things that may appear to be random listings are in a particular order for distinct reasons. Revelation came suddenly and as a question, "I wonder if the order of the days of creation has anything to do with our health?"

I dropped the mop, ran to my Bible, opened to Genesis 1, and began praising God. There in the first chapter of the Bible God's design for perfect health was revealed. The days of creation are listed according to the priority of their importance to our health and wholeness. Decades of research by modern nutritionists and scientists are verifying God's Word, written thousands of years ago! Isn't that amazing?

God's Balance and Purpose in Creation

Balance and purpose are evident throughout creation. God's order of creation can be separated into two triads. The days listed in each triad are in exact order according to what is most beneficial to our health and well being. These two triads explicitly show us how to live healthy, balanced, purposeful lives.

The triads are as follows:

Triads of Creation

Triad #1		Triad #2	
Day One:	Light (happiness)	**Fourth Day:**	Sun, Moon and Stars
Second Day:	Air	**Fifth Day:**	Fish
	Water		Fowl
Third Day:	Land	**Sixth Day:**	Animals
	Plants		Man

Seventh Day: Sabbath Rest

Not only are the creations of the first triad directly related to the creations of the second triad, but they also had to be in place to sustain the creations of the second triad. The creations of the two triads directly correspond to each other.

- The Light (**Day One**) had to exist for the lights of the sun, moon, and stars (**Fourth Day**) to receive it.
- Air and Water (**Second Day**) had to exist to provide a place for Fish and Fowl (**Fifth Day**) to live. (If it appears to you that fish and fowl should be reversed due to the order of their respective abodes—air and water—remember that everything is listed in the exact order according to what is most beneficial to our health. This will be discussed later in greater detail.)

- Land and Plant life **(Third Day)** had to exist so Animals and Man **(Sixth Day)** could survive.
- Sabbath Rest **(Seventh Day)** completed the cycle by bringing the emphasis of all creation back to the Creator.

The remaining chapters of this book will examine each day of creation separately to illustrate its relation to our total well being. God used balance and purpose in His process of creating the world. Isn't that amazing?

NUTRITIONAL APPLICATION

BALANCE AND ORDER

For the life of a creature is in the blood, and I have given it to you to make atonement for yourselves on the altar; it is the blood that makes atonement for one's life (Leviticus 17:11).

Thousands of years ago God gave the following truth: the secret to life is in the blood. The body is made of approximately one hundred trillion cells, according to researchers. Each cell is a living, functional organism. An individual cell moves, breathes, takes in food, digests, excretes, and reproduces. To remain healthy, a cell must receive proper nourishment and toxins must be removed.

How does this happen? It happens through the blood! The main purposes of the blood are to deliver life-giving nutrients to the cell and to remove toxins for excretion. When this happens, a person is healthy. When this does not happen, a person is sick.

Homeostasis

Balance is the key to health. In 1932, Dr. Walter B. Cannon authored a book entitled The Wisdom of the Body. In it he used the word "homeostasis," which described the electro-magnetic and chemical balances of the body. In recent years the importance of homeostasis in the body has been acclaimed as crucial to good health.

The body is comprised of 68% oxygen. Oxygen is delivered to the cells through the blood system. When the body is in homeostasis, the acid-alkaline condition (pH) is balanced. On a scale of 0-14, seven is considered balanced. Although most of the fluids of the body are alkaline, the bodily functions produce acidity in the body. Alkaline blood is able to carry more oxygen to the cells and the presence of oxygen hinders the growth of germs. Therefore, the proper pH balance of the body is necessary for healthy living.

Balance in Nutrients

Another important fact about balance is that the nutrients in the body work in relation to each other. For example, water, carbohydrates, fats, proteins, and vitamins, as well as micronutrients, enzymes, and amino acids are dependent on minerals for their proper functioning. If the body is in homeostasis, these elements work synergistically (in unity) with each other.

However, when the body is not in balance it can either produce an over abundance of some nutrients causing toxicity, or a shortage that renders other nutrients useless or ineffective. It all depends on balance.

Circadian Rhythms and Cycles of the Body

The body functions according to set patterns of rhythms and cycles. Even the most basic activities of the body perform in ways that are orderly and balanced.

The rhythms of the body are called the circadian rhythms. This term is a combination of the Latin words *circa* meaning "around, near, or close to" and *dias* meaning "day." The British chronobiologist, Josephine Arendt, once wrote, "Everything is rhythmic unless proved otherwise."

Cycles in the body occur over varying periods of time. Some of these cycles are as follows:

Digestive Rhythms

The rhythm of the body concerning the digestion, absorption, and elimination of food is balanced. It is agreed generally that this process is divided into the following three eight-hour cycles:

Elimination—From 4:00 a.m. to 12:00 noon. the body is in a cleansing mode, removing waste materials from the body. You may have noticed that you feel the need to eliminate more frequently in the morning.

Appropriation—Between 12:00 noon and 8:00 p.m. the body is in a cycle where eating and digestion of food are taking place.

Assimilation—From 8:00 p.m. to 4:00 a.m. the body is absorbing the nutrients from the previously digested food.

Circadian Rhythms of the Body

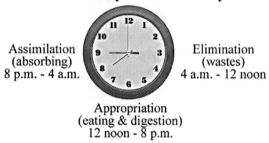

Assimilation
(absorbing)
8 p.m. - 4 a.m.

Elimination
(wastes)
4 a.m. - 12 noon

Appropriation
(eating & digestion)
12 noon - 8 p.m.

This cycle is important for us to heed concerning our dietary habits. It is best not to eat after 8:00 p.m. Food consumed after that time diverts the body's energy from assimilation to digestion.

Light/Dark, Day/Night Cycle

Our bodies have internal clocks that tell us when to awaken, when to sleep, and even when to begin to prepare for sleep. We sleep and wake up best when we heed the rhythm of our internal clocks.

Every morning before a person awakens his or her body temperature and blood pressure rise. In addition, the heart beats faster and glands squirt pulses of hormones needed for bodily activity.

At night, the opposite occurs. The body temperature, blood pressure and heart rate fall. Sleep hormones are increased and those needed for bodily activity are lowered.

Menstrual Cycle

A woman's menstruation occurs in a twenty-eight day cycle. This cycle coincides with the lunar calendar, upon which the Bible's religious observances are based.

In addition, a man's beard grows during a seven-day cycle. All the rhythms and cycles of the body are developed to perform in an orderly way. Once again, balance is the key. Isn't that amazing?

Balance and Health

The secret of staying healthy, or regaining health, can be found in the order and balance of the days of the creation week.

DAYS OF CREATION	
Day 1	**Light and Happiness** A relationship with the Creator produces inner happiness and joy.
2nd Day	**Air** Adequate oxygen is needed by the body. Deep breathing and moderate exercise promote oxygenation. **Water** Sufficient water intake daily (8 ounces per 20 pounds of body weight) is vital.
3rd Day	**Earth** **Plant Life** Vegetables, seeds (including nuts, whole grains, legumes), and fruits are the most nutritious foods. They transfer minerals from the earth to the beings who eat them.
4th Day	**Sun, Moon, and Stars** Moderate sunlight, ample sleep, meaningful religious observances, seasonal foods, and graceful maturity promote health.
5th Day	**Fish** **Fowl** If one chooses to eat meat, fish is the most healthful, and fowl is second.
6th Day	**Animals** Biblical dietary laws govern the following foods: Livestock (cattle) is permissible (herbivorous and/or granivorous). Creeping animals are forbidden (carnivorous). Wild animals are forbidden (carnivorous). **Man** Man has a free will to make beneficial lifestyle choices.
7th Day	**Sabbath Rest** The Sabbath offers time to reflect on God and experience holiness, rest, and joy.

God made it simple when He gave us the formula for health. He even revealed it in the order of what is most beneficial for us. Isn't that amazing?

The True "Circle of Life"

The term "circle of life" has become quite popular in recent times. Amazingly, God established the true circle of life when He created the world.

God, the Master Architect, could have designed the earth in any shape He desired. However, in His wisdom, He carefully selected a circle (sphere) as the earth's shape. Remember, there is purpose to everything that God does.

Not only did He create the world to be a circle, in looking clockwise, the elements of the days of creation form a circle. It can be considered circular because the order of creation **begins and ends with God!**

The Circle of Life

Light
(Happiness)

Sabbath

Air, Water

Animals, Man

Fish, Fowl

Dry Land,
Vegetation

Sun, Moon, and Stars

God showed us from the dawn of creation how to live balanced lives. In the process, He incorporated provisions for the spirit, soul, and body. However, God gave us the choice of whether or not to accept His provisions and live according to His intended balance. Isn't that amazing?

Satan's Efforts to Destroy God's Balance of Creation

God longs for us to live healthy, happy, purposeful lives as He has shown through His Word. Our gracious God wants us not only to live, but to live abundantly.

However, the Bible teaches that there is an enemy, Satan, who is out to destroy all of God's creations. Satan knows that if we are imbalanced in spirit, soul, and body, we cannot accomplish what our Creator put us on earth to do. Satan wants us to live weak, sickly lives and die without having fulfilled our purposes in life. John 10:10 states that *the thief* [ultimately Satan] *comes only to steal, and kill, and destroy: I* [Jesus] *have come that they might have life, and have it to the full.*

God has given us the freedom to choose lifestyles that will keep our total beings in balance. This is God's desire for us. However, we also have the freedom to choose lifestyles that will destroy the balance of our total being. This is Satan's desire for us.

It is no coincidence that the first temptation centered around a lifestyle choice involving food (Genesis 3:1-7). Adam and Eve were allowed to eat the fruit of every tree in the garden—except one—the tree of the knowledge of good and evil. Satan convinced them to eat the forbidden fruit, and his tactics are no different today. Daily, he tempts us to eat harmful foods and make lifestyle choices contrary to what is best for us. Why do we, like Adam and Eve, continue to fall for his deception?

Choices that Diminish the Benefits of Balance and Order

Imbalance and Disease

In 1992, the National Center for Health Statistics reported that 70% of all deaths in the United States are the result of heart disease or cancer. It was further reported that 80% of those deaths could have been prevented by lifestyle changes. That is a sobering statistic.

When the body is not in homeostasis and the pH balance is upset, free radical damage is more likely to occur. Pairs of electrons exist in the nuclei of cells. When sugar and oxygen are converted into energy, these pairs of electrons can lose a partner. Cells that have lost an electron partner are called free radicals.

In an attempt to stabilize themselves, the cells seek to steal electrons from other nuclei. This results in a chain reaction in the body that causes cellular chaos and attributes greatly to disease in the body. When the body is balanced, the immune system is able to keep this process under control. When the body is imbalanced, the immune system is suppressed and free radical damage results in sickness and disease.

Toxic Overload of the Immune System

Every day within our bodies billions of cells die and are replaced by new ones. This process produces toxins within the body. Ordinarily, the body's amazing immune system can handle the toxins. The lymph system, the main component of the immune system, cleanses the toxins and carries them away from the tissues. However, disease results when toxins placed into the body through poor lifestyle choices combine with toxins produced by bodily functions to exceed what the immune system can handle.

If we choose imbalanced lifestyles, we rob ourselves of good health. We also bring on premature aging and death, which is exactly what Satan wants.

A NEW BEGINNING

Sometimes It Gets Worse Before It Gets Better

A principle in life seems to be that things often get worse before they get better. For example, darkness precedes light, and sorrow precedes joy. When we decide to improve our health through lifestyle changes, we usually go through a time called a "healing crisis." As we abandon a diet of harmful substances and replace it with life-giving foods, our bodies experience a detoxification period.

Detoxification symptoms vary from mild to severe, depending upon the person and his or her previous degree of bodily abuse. Detoxification symptoms include fatigue, headaches, upset stomachs, aching muscles, sore throats and/or congestion.

Generally, detoxification symptoms are short-lived. Some may only last a few hours while others may remain for a few days, or in severe cases, weeks. Try to keep focused on the fact that this is a "healing crisis" and that, like any other crisis, it will pass with time. People often become discouraged during detoxification and return to former lifestyles before they give their bodies enough time to regain health.

God designed us in such a way that our bodies long to be healthy. Health is the innate goal of each body. Our bodies respond positively to every step we take toward that goal.

Therefore, we must not give up. Our bodies did not become

tired, overweight, and unhealthy overnight, but rather over a period of time. Keep in mind that it will also take a period of time to return to good health.

SPIRITUAL APPLICATION

Spirit, Soul, and Body

According to biblical Hebrew thought, our Creator designed us with three aspects that interrelate to produce who we are as individuals. Each is dependent upon the other to produce "us." Although each is distinct, the three cannot be separated. They are as follows:

Spirit—our loftiest part by which we are able to commune with God
Soul—our mental and emotional make-up, the essence of who we are
Body—our physical component

We are made in the *image* and *likeness* of God—spirit, soul and body. One facet of this truth is that we are like the persons of the Godhead who are One, yet each has distinctive characteristics. One does not exist without the other. God the Father, God the Son, and God the Holy Spirit exist as a unit.

The same is true of us as individuals. The spirit (spiritual), soul (mental and emotional), and body (physical) are one, yet each has distinctive characteristics. One does not exist without the other. The spirit, soul, and body exist as a unit.

The spirit (spiritual) is in the *likeness* of God, the Holy Spirit. His characteristics are available also to those who have received His indwelling: *But the fruit of the Spirit is love, joy, peace, patience, kindness, goodness, faithfulness, gentleness, and self-control. . .* (Galatians 5:22-23).

The soul (mental and emotional) is in the *likeness* of God the Father. God's heart is filled with a variety of emotions toward His creations, especially love: *Dear friends, let us love one another, for love comes from God* (I John 4:7). However, we also are told in scripture that there are times when He experiences anger: *The wrath of God is being revealed from heaven against all the godless-*

ness and wickedness of men who suppress the truth by their wickedness (Romans 1:18), and even jealousy: *. . for I, the Lord your God, am a jealous God. . .* (Exodus 20:5).

The body (physical) is in the *image* of Jesus, who was the bodily form of God on earth: *The Word became flesh and made his dwelling among us* (John 1:14). *And being found in appearance as a man, He humbled Himself and became obedient to death—even death on a cross!* (Philippians 2:8)

Isn't it wonderful to be made in God's likeness and image? Only mankind has this distinction.

It is exciting to realize that when a person accepts the gift of Jesus' atoning sacrifice on the cross his or her spirit is reborn. This new birth makes one a child of God and assures eternal life in His presence. The spirit is made righteous through Christ: *But if Christ is in you, your body is dead because of sin, yet your spirit is alive because of righteousness* (Romans 8:10).

It is exciting also to realize that when we are in God's presence in heaven we will have a new mind and heart (soul): *When he appears, we shall be like him, for we shall see him as he is* (I John 3:2).

We will also have a new body, a perfect body: *The body that is sown is perishable, it is raised imperishable; it is sown in dishonor, it is raised in glory; it is sown in weakness, it is raised in power; it is sown a natural body, it is raised a spiritual body* (I Corinthians 15:42-44).

Thus, from the beginning of the creation narrative, we sense God's balance of spirit, soul, and body for each person. If we follow the blueprint concealed in the creation story, our lives will be balanced. The order of the days of creation adequately provides for each dimension.

God gave man dominion over all living things on the earth, thereby allowing him to choose those from which he could benefit. He created us with the privilege and responsibility of making the right lifestyle choices.

The heart of the matter is that balance in the spirit, soul, and body can be acquired by the following:

1) A relationship with the Creator resulting in inner happiness and joy

2) Adequate oxygen (which deep breathing and moderate exercise enhance)
3) Sufficient water intake
4) Diet consisting primarily of vegetation
5) Sunlight, ample rest, religious observances, seasonal foods, graceful aging
6) Limited intake of meat and animal products
7) A time to reflect on God and experience rest, holiness and joy

Choosing to live in relationship with the Giver of life will empower us to make the choices that benefit us and glorify Him. He truly is *the beginning and the ending* (Revelation 1:8 KJV), and *the author and perfecter of our faith* (Hebrews 12:2).

I recently heard someone say, "God gives the test before He teaches the lesson." This is confirmed in Isaiah 46:10, when God said that He will *make known the end from the beginning*.

Many of us have failed the test. Our imbalanced lives are the evidence. However, for students who are willing to learn the lessons, there is hope. His love allows us to re-test. It is an open book test and He has given us the answers already. They can be found in Genesis 1:1 through Genesis 2:3.

Throughout this chapter I have concluded sections with the phrase "Isn't that amazing?" When we consider God's awesome plan of creation and His tender care in preserving the balance of life, truly it is amazing!

Dear God,

Thank You for creating a beautifully balanced world. Thank You for creating me to live in that world. Help me make the choices that will glorify You and benefit my health. I desire to accomplish the purposes for which You created me. Please guide me as I commit to do so.

In Jesus' name I pray, Amen.

MEMORY VERSE FOR *IN THE BEGINNING*:
May your whole spirit, soul, and body be kept blameless at the coming of our Lord Jesus Christ (I Thessalonians 5:23b).

ASSIGNMENT(S) FOR *IN THE BEGINNING*:

1) Prayerfully consider your lifestyle. **Identify things that are out of balance in your life.** Into which category do they fall— spirit, soul, or body?

2) With God's help, **list positive steps** you can take to make the necessary changes.

DEVOTIONAL FOR *IN THE BEGINNING*

Day One

Scripture Reading: Luke 2:40-52

Verse of the Day: *And Jesus grew in wisdom and stature, and in favor with God and men* (Luke 2:52).

Jesus has been and always will be the perfect role model. This verse gives the formula for patterning our lives after His. Luke informs us that Jesus led a balanced life. Jesus grew mentally (in wisdom), physically (in stature), spiritually (in favor with God), and emotionally (in favor with men). In other words, He grew in spirit (spiritually), soul (mentally and emotionally), and body (physically). As His followers, we are to endeavor to do the same.

Often we put emphasis on one of these areas to the neglect of the others. The result is a life out of balance. For example, people who are obsessed with physical fitness may neglect the expansion of their minds through continual learning. Others may be so studious or work-oriented that they become recluses, avoiding people. However, the greatest tragedy is when any emphasis leads to the neglect of developing a personal relationship with God.

Once while driving my car on a routine errand, the steering wheel suddenly began to shake. At first it only shook a little, but continued to worsen until it was difficult to keep the car on the road. I stopped by a service station and the mechanic discovered that the front tires were out of balance. Just one part of the car out of balance had affected the entire car, making it almost impossible to drive.

The same is true of our lives. One unbalanced area can affect dramatically the other parts of our lives, causing us to lose sight of our reasons for living. As with Jesus, we find our purposes in life as we develop a balance among spirit, soul, and body.

Application:
1) If there is an area of your life (spirit, soul, or body) that is out of balance, are you aware of the reason(s) it has become so?
2) What is one positive step you can take to bring more balance to that area?

PRAY for guidance to follow the example of Jesus and maintain balance in your life.

DEVOTIONAL FOR *IN THE BEGINNING*

Day Two

Scripture Reading: Proverbs 3:13-24

Verse of the Day: *Blessed is the man who finds wisdom, and the man who gains understanding* (Proverbs 3:13).

Jesus grew in wisdom (Luke 2:52). Growing mentally is an exciting adventure. I read of a mother who asked her first grade child what he had learned in school that day. He replied, "I learned things I didn't understand and then I learned to understand them." What a priceless explanation of learning!

Solomon wrote in Proverbs that when we are balanced in the area of mental growth (wisdom), we find happiness. He also states, in Proverbs 3:16, that being balanced can help prolong our lives. Scientists have proven that one of the strongest deterrents to the aging process is learning. As long as the brain is processing new information, the aging process slows significantly. How amazing that God, through Solomon, had told us that fact thousands of years ago! Failing to think new thoughts and gain more knowledge is like living, eating, and sleeping in only one room of a mansion.

Solomon also declares, *the fear of the Lord is the beginning of wisdom, and knowledge of the Holy One is understanding* (Proverbs 9:10). In biblical Hebrew, the word *fear* actually means "reverence." Therefore, we can see clearly that the process of becoming mentally balanced begins with a relationship with the Creator of all wisdom.

Application:

1) Do you feel that you make an effort to grow mentally?
2) How many books do you read each year? Do they include a variety of topics?
3) How often do you read God's Word? Do you study the Bible and apply it, or merely read the words?
4) If change is needed in this area of your life, how do you intend to bring about the change?

PRAY for strength to stay close to God so you can grow mentally as you learn from the Source of all knowledge.

DEVOTIONAL FOR *IN THE BEGINNING*

Day Three

Scripture Reading: Psalm 139:1-24

Verse of the Day: *Therefore, I urge you, brothers, in view of God's mercy, to offer your bodies as living sacrifices, holy and pleasing to God—this is your spiritual act of worship* (Romans 12:1).

Jesus grew in stature (Luke 2:52). The human body is intricately, yet delicately designed. As the psalmist declared, *"I will praise you because I am fearfully and wonderfully made"* (Psalm 139:14).

When our older daughter was a young child, she ran into the kitchen one day and asked with wide-eyed exuberance, "How come when you move your feet you go places?" Have you ever tried to explain the process of walking to a child? Each aspect of our bodies is so astounding, I find myself living in the same state of amazement that our daughter expressed.

Recently, a friend shared that her husband had quoted laughingly the late George Burns' statement, "If I had known I would live this long, I would have taken better care of myself." Although he made the statement in jest, he spoke a profound truth. God has given each of us a body to house our souls. Our bodies have to last a lifetime, so we must care for them with wisdom and tenderness.

Many times we simply do not realize how precious our physical health is until we encounter sickness or disease. I read the following verse in a very old book I found in the library:

> *To get his wealth he spent his health,*
> *And then with might and main*
> *He turned around and spent his wealth*
> *To get his health again*
> (Golden Treasury).

Paul reminds us in our scripture for today that we are expected to present our bodies as a living sacrifice to God. A *living sacrifice* means we will have to give up some things in order to accomplish this. But, as Paul also reminds us, our bodies are the temple of God and really belong to Him anyway: *Do you not know that your body is a temple of the Holy Spirit. . . ?* (I Corinthians 6:19) What kind of custodians of His temple are we?

Application:
1) Are you presenting your body as a living sacrifice to God?
2) If not, what do you need to change in order to do so?
3) What would God have you do as the first step in becoming more balanced physically?

PRAY and thank God for the wonderful way He created you.

DEVOTIONAL FOR *IN THE BEGINNING*

Day Four

Scripture Reading: Hebrews 11:1-40

Verse of the Day: *And without faith it is impossible to please God, because anyone who comes to him must believe that he exists and that he rewards those who earnestly seek him* (Hebrews 11:6).

Jesus grew in favor with God (Luke 2:52). Our verse of the day reveals how we can grow in favor with God. The secret to keeping our spiritual lives in balance is faith, and more specifically, faith in God. Without faith it is impossible to please or "find favor with" God.

For our faith to be grounded, we must focus on <u>Who</u> God is and not <u>what</u> He is doing. God is always the same, never changing! However, His methods may change according to what is most beneficial for each believer. He always does what is best for His children. When we truly realize that, we can develop a faith that leads to complete trust in Him.

As earthly parents we may love each of our children equally, but do for them in different ways according to the personality, the needs, and the circumstances of each child. In a much larger sense, the same is true of God. Some people lose faith when they look at what is happening in the lives of others and wonder why God is not doing the same things for them. However, we can rest assured that, if we allow Him, God will work in our lives in the ways that are best for us.

We must stay focused on God and His precious promises. He is holy, just, pure, loving, fair, merciful, wise, and, yes, balanced! Truly believing this is the way we can stay balanced spiritually.

Helen Keller, the noted deaf and blind author and lecturer once wrote the following:

Dark as my path may seem to others,
I carry a magic light in my heart.
Faith, the spiritual strong searchlight illumines the way.

Although sinister doubts lurk in the shadow,
I walk unafraid toward the Enchanted Wood
      where the foliage is always green; where joy abides;
where nightingales nest and sing,
      and where life and death are one
in the presence of the Lord.

Application:
1) Is your faith strong enough to be pleasing to God?
2) What causes you to doubt?
3) How can you become balanced spiritually?

PRAY for faith to trust God in all circumstances.

DEVOTIONAL FOR *IN THE BEGINNING*

Day Five

Scripture Reading: I Corinthians 13:1-13

Verse of the Day: *But if we walk in the light, as he is in the light, we have fellowship with one another, and the blood of Jesus, his Son, purifies us from all sin* (I John 1:7).

Jesus grew in favor with men (Luke 2:52). John explains how to become socially balanced. It is a natural result of walking in the light. *Walk in the light* simply means obeying the commandments of God.

While He was on earth, friendship was very important to Jesus. There are many accounts of His social interactions. He attended a wedding party (Cana); He stayed in the home of friends (Mary, Martha, and Lazarus); He ate in the home of friends (Matthew and Zacchaeus); and He observed special feasts and holidays with friends (Passover).

Jesus loved His friends and they knew it. He not only shared happy occasions with them, He also shared sad experiences with them. When He heard Lazarus was seriously ill, Jesus went to Mary and Martha's home. Upon learning of Lazarus' death, He cried with them (John 11:35).

Jesus was always there for His friends. When they needed Him, He was available. Once, when the disciples were in a storm at sea in the middle of the night, He walked across the water to get to them (Matthew 14:25).

Jesus forgave His friends. Peter denied Jesus three times before the crucifixion. After His resurrection, Jesus gave Peter three chances to relieve the guilt of denying Him (John 21:15-17).

From Jesus' example we find the true meaning of friendship. Through friendship we become balanced socially and grow *in favor with men*. Robert Louis Stevenson once penned that "a friend is a present you give yourself." Are you willing to give yourself that present?

Application:
1) Who is your best friend?
2) What makes that friendship so special?
3) Do you give more or take more in the relationship?
4) What steps can you take to become more balanced socially?

PRAY for the ability to be a friend like Jesus.

DEVOTIONAL FOR *IN THE BEGINNING*

Day Six

Scripture Reading: Romans 7:7-25

Verse of the Day: *But seek first his kingdom and his righteousness, and all these things will be given to you as well* (Matthew 6:33).

The secret to living a balanced life mentally, physically, spiritually, and socially boils down to one thing—PRIORITIES. Dr. William Mitchell, noted author and lecturer, explains that "God doesn't make winners or losers, He makes choosers."

When considering a career choice, one of our daughters exclaimed to me, "I don't like making all these decisions." I replied, "That's what life is...a series of decisions." We often remind our children that each person has to live with the consequences of his or her choices.

This is true as we consider how important it is for us to keep our lives in balance. Everyone has the same number of hours in a day. No one has any more or any less than another person. How we use those hours is up to us. To stay in balance, we must make choices that will promote spiritual, mental, physical, and social health.

David Starr Jordan stated, "Be a life long or short, its completeness depends on what it was lived for." In his poem The Arrow, Henry Van Dyke wrote the following:

> *Life is an arrow—therefore you must know*
>   *what mark to aim at,*
> *how to use the bow—then draw it to the head and let it go.*

God has given us the bow and the instructions to use it. Whether or not we aim at the mark is up to us. How do we achieve balance in our lives? Seek first His kingdom—and all these things will be given to you as well.

Application:
1) Set one priority for this week.
2) Write it down, and share it with a friend who will hold you accountable.
3) Commit to accomplish it with God's help.

PRAY and thank God for providing help as you grow spiritually, mentally, physically, and socially.

DEVOTIONAL FOR *IN THE BEGINNING*

Day Seven

Scripture Reading: I Thessalonians 5:1-28

Verse of the Day: *May God himself, the God of peace, sanctify you* *through and through. May your whole spirit, and soul and body be kept blameless at the coming of our Lord Jesus Christ* (I Thessalonians 5:23).

This chapter is both powerful and practical. Paul admonishes the early church in I Thessalonians 5:1-11 that, in *the day of the Lord* (v.2), Jesus will come to receive those who are "sanctified" to live with Him. The Greek word used here for *sanctify* is *hagiazo,* which means "to purify, to make holy." He warns believers to remain holy and on guard for this moment, for it will come *like a thief in the night* (v.4).

Paul continues with a checklist of succinct, yet profound, ways to live *sanctified* lives and to remain ready for this glorious event. The list is as follows:

- ✔ respect church leaders and spiritual gifts within the congregation (vs.12,13; 20)
- ✔ keep peace and unity (v.13)
- ✔ help those who are rebellious, mentally challenged, and physically challenged (v.14)
- ✔ practice patience and avoid revenge (vs.14,15)
- ✔ do good and evade even the appearance of evil (vs.15, 21, 22)
- ✔ rejoice with "an attitude of gratitude" (vs.16,18)
- ✔ pray constantly (v.17)
- ✔ discern right from wrong (v.21)
- ✔ do not quench the Spirit of God (v.19).

Only the blood of Jesus can purify us. However, once we have been cleansed by Him, Paul's advice can help us live *sanctified* lives in spirit, soul and body.

According to Jewish tradition, when a couple became "betrothed," similar to engagement, the bride was required to wear a veil over her face in public. The veil indicated that she had been "set apart" for her future bridegroom. In this way she demonstrated that she was remaining pure for him and loyal to him.

Likewise, as those who await our Bridegroom, Jesus Christ, we are to be "set apart." Our lives should demonstrate that we are remaining pure for Him and loyal to Him. Even the strength to be "set apart" for Him comes from Him: *The one who calls you is faithful and he will do it* (I Thessalonians 5:24).

<u>Application</u>:
1) Reflect on the above checklist and decide which disciplines you practice faithfully.
2) Reflect on the above checklist and decide which ones you neglect, or even ignore.
3) Place the list in a prominent place so you can remind yourself that you are to be sanctified in preparation for the coming of the Lord.

PRAY and ask God to help you live in such a way that it is obvious you belong to Him. Thank God that the strength to live for Him also comes from Him.

CHAPTER ONE

BIBLICAL APPLICATION

Day One of Creation

(Genesis 1:1-5)

1 In the beginning God created the heavens and the earth. 2 Now the earth was formless and empty, darkness was over the surface of the deep, and the Spirit of God was hovering over the waters. 3 And God said, "Let there be light," and there was light. 4 God saw that the light was good, and he separated the light from the darkness. 5 God called the light "day," and the darkness he called "night." And there was evening, and there was morning—the first day [in the original Hebrew it is referred to as "day one"].

LIGHT (HAPPINESS)

The dawn of creation—day one in the history of the world—is recorded in the opening chapter of the Bible. On day one God created heaven and earth. The Hebrew word for *created* used in this opening verse of the Bible is *bara* indicating "to create out of nothing."

Genesis tells us that the newly created heaven and earth were *formless* and *empty*. Neither heaven nor earth acquired their present forms until a later day of creation.

From Genesis 1:2 it appears that the mass of earth and the atmosphere were co-mingled in some type of shapeless liquid. The earth was dark, formless, watery, and possibly unattractive. Yet God knew His intention from the very beginning. He saw beyond what it was to what it would become! God had a plan for this shapeless mass. He had a purpose.

The Spirit of God hovered over the waters. The Hebrew phrase used for *Spirit of God* is *Ruach Elohim*, which means "Breath of the Strong and Mighty One." The very breath of God began fashioning beauty out of emptiness.

Then, through the power of His Word, creation proceeded. God summoned light into existence with the mere words, *let there be light,* or literally, "let light be." How simple, yet how profound this is! Prior to the introduction of light, the newly created world was shrouded in darkness. It is extremely important that we comprehend this. The world was dark until God called forth light into existence.

This light was not the light given by the sun, moon, and stars, for those celestial objects were not created until the fourth day. The light referred to in this passage is a different light.

In the physical sense, this light was indicative of God infusing the world with radiant physical energy. However, throughout scripture, God uses the physical to hint at, or to point to, a spiritual meaning. This scripture is a perfect example as the Hebrew word for *light* shows a deeper, spiritual meaning.

The Hebrew word used here for *light* is *owr*, which means "illumination." It also means "happiness." How like God that is! Before He continued creating the world, He bathed it in His light and happiness. His intention from the beginning was that all creation live in this light and happiness.

An understanding of, and relationship with, the Creator of this light, is the very core of <u>The Creation Diet</u>. Living a balanced, healthy life is a spiritual matter. This light, in the spiritual sense, is representative of God.

The Hebrew word, *owr* (light and happiness), is used throughout the Old Testament. It often refers to the following:

Light in Scripture

- The presence of God .... (Isaiah 60:19, 20)
- The guidance of God .... (Exodus 13:21; 14:20)
- The revelation of God .... (Isaiah 2:5; Micah 7:8)
- The Word of God .... (Psalm 119:105; 119:130)
- The judgment of God .... (Zephaniah 3:5; Hosea 6:5)

Furthermore, in the New Testament we read that *God is light; in him there is no darkness* (I John 1:5). Jesus also proclaimed in John 8:32 that He is the light of the world, and those who trust in Him are children of the *light* (John 12:36).

From these passages, as well as from many others throughout scripture, the correlation between God's light and true happiness becomes apparent. Scripture repeatedly states that those who trust in the Lord are happy (Psalm 84:5; 146:5; Proverbs 16:20; 28:14; Jeremiah 17:7; Revelation 14:3; 19:9; 22:14). It is imperative to understand that a relationship with God is the starting point toward a happy, healthy, balanced life.

Why is this true? The answer is because only God can give the wisdom to make the choices that are best for our lives. In addition, only He can give us the strength to live consistently by those choices.

In contrast, throughout the Bible darkness is equated with the following:

Darkness in Scripture

- Lack of understanding ... (Psalm 82:5; Ecclesiastes 2:14)
- Wrong choices .... (Proverbs 12:13)
- Sorrow .... (Joel 2:2; Zephaniah 1:15)
- Blindness .... (I John 2:11; Luke 11:34)
- Sin .... (Romans 13:12-14)
- Hell .... (Matthew 22:13; Revelation 16:10)

Walking in the light means that we trust and obey God. Walking in darkness means that we doubt and disobey Him.

NUTRITIONAL APPLICATION

I. SPIRITUAL LIGHT

Many physicians now emphasize that spiritual beliefs are a major factor in wellness. Doctors have stated that patients who believe in God have a much higher cure rate than those who believe their lives will end when their bodies die.

Over 200 studies in medical journals report that prayer and spirituality make a person healthier. In fact, a recent government-sponsored survey found that 43% of doctors admit that they pray for their patients.

In 1998, an interesting experiment took place at San Francisco General Hospital. Under the guidance of cardiologist Randolph Byrd, 393 patients were studied over a ten-month period. Half of the patients were selected randomly to receive intercessory prayer by several religious groups. The other half was not assigned for prayer by anyone.

The astounding results were that, in the group with members who had been prayed for, fewer patients died. They had significantly fewer complications and were five times less likely to need antibiotics. None required ventilation to assist breathing. The group that did not receive intercessory prayer experienced more deaths and significant complications. Twelve patients of that group had to be placed on ventilation.

Duke University Medical Center conducted a project that focused on 1,700 older Americans. The results of the study showed that those who attended religious services had a stronger immune system than those who did not. About 60% of those in the study, both men and women, attended religious services at least once a week. Their blood tests showed that they were less likely to have high levels of a certain protein that is linked to diseases associated with aging.

The previous study did not prove conclusively whether people were healthier as a result of attending worship regularly or if they worshipped regularly because they were healthy. However, earlier studies had confirmed a correlation between good health and the observance of religious standards and traditions. Honoring God does have positive effects on health.

CHOICES THAT DIMINISH THE BENEFITS OF LIGHT

In the previous chapter it was established that whether or not we live a balanced life is a matter of choice. The same is true of whether we choose to walk in light or darkness.

Jesus said, *"This is the verdict: light has come into the world, but men loved darkness instead of light because their deeds were evil"* (John 3:19). God's light will lead us in the ways that ensure happy, healthy lives. Satan will lead us away from those things. The choice is simple — darkness or light. Which will we choose?

II. HAPPINESS

As stated previously, the connotation of the Hebrew word, *owr*, is more than merely "light." It also means "happiness." God's first desire for us is that we know Him as the Source of light, and be filled with inner happiness.

The importance of happiness in relation to a healthy body was addressed succinctly, yet profoundly, by King Solomon in Proverbs 17:22. He stated simply, *"A cheerful heart is good medicine, but a crushed spirit dries up the bones."* Solomon knew that there is a definite relation between the mind and the body. A cheerful heart *is* good medicine.

Humor Therapy

Perhaps the greatest example that a cheerful heart is good medicine comes from Norman Cousins. Over twenty years ago, Cousins had an autoimmune disease called *ankylosing spondylitis*. This disease is a life-threatening form of arthritis that attacks the connective tissues. He became crippled, and he experienced severe pain constantly. In spite of what seemed like a hopeless situation, Cousins found a way to thwart the disease and bring himself back to health. How did he do it?

Norman Cousins began taking massive doses of Vitamin C and

laughing himself well. Yes, that is right, <u>laughing</u> himself well! He watched hour after hour of "Marx Brothers" films, reruns of "Candid Camera" and old "I Love Lucy" shows. According to Cousins, ten minutes of hearty laughter lowered his pain level for two hours. He later wrote about his unusual self-prescribed therapy in <u>Anatomy of an Illness</u>. Although he did not have a medical background, he became an adjunct professor of psychiatry at UCLA's Medical School. Cousins is considered the father of humor therapy, but that distinction should be attributed to God. It was He who first bathed the world in light and happiness.

Physical Benefits of Laughter

Since laughter (or at least a smile) is an outer manifestation of happiness, it is important to understand some physical benefits of laughter. First of all, laughter is a good workout. It gives the muscles of your face, shoulders, diaphragm, and abdomen much needed exercise. Norman Cousins calls laughter "inner jogging."

As with any exercise, during and immediately following laughter the heart rate and blood pressure rise temporarily. Breathing becomes faster and deeper causing life-giving oxygen to surge through the bloodstream.

In addition, laughter strengthens the immune system. It boosts antibodies in saliva. It also increases white blood cells and immunoglobulin A, which are disease-fighting immune cells. At the same time, laughter decreases stress chemicals, such as cortisol and epinephrine, which suppress the immune system.

A wonderful result of laughter is that it reduces stress. It increases the body's production of chemicals in the brain known as endorphins. Endorphins, especially seratonin, give the body a heightened sense of well being, and serve as pain relievers. Taking all of this into consideration, it is no wonder King Solomon declared thousands of years ago that *a cheerful heart is good medicine* (Proverbs 17:22).

Thanks to Norman Cousins and the research that followed his recovery, modern science has developed laughter medicine as a therapeutic way of dealing with illness. It involves the three steps of stretching, laughing, and being silent. King Solomon would be proud!

CHOICES THAT DIMINISH THE BENEFITS OF HAPPINESS

Have you ever considered the fact that humans are the only creatures who have the ability to laugh? Ordinarily, babies begin to laugh when they are around ten weeks old. Approximately six weeks later, they are laughing once each hour. By the age of four, they are laughing once every four minutes. However, the average adult in America laughs only about fifteen times a day. What happens to cause this decrease in laughter?

Daily our lives are filled with obstacles that cause stress and frustration. Among these are illness, financial strain, relationship problems with family, friends, and/or co-workers, and job dissatisfaction. Psychologists tell us that 80% of what we experience daily is negative. Also, 90% of what we tell ourselves mentally is negative. Happiness is enhanced when we filter the negative and allow only what is beneficial to enter our minds.

This is a constant and continuous process—thought by thought. Our thought patterns are some of Satan's most effective tools to keep us in bondage and darkness. Our thoughts evoke emotions that lead to behavior. Our behaviors over a period of time become our habits, and our habits eventually produce our character. (Thoughts + emotions + behavior + habits = character.)

Replacement Therapy

In her book, Untie the Ribbons, Sharon Hoffman examines the importance of Replacement Therapy. (Not to be confused with Hormone Replacement Therapy.) Sharon advocates using Replacement Therapy to combat negative thoughts. When a negative thought, which is usually a lie from Satan, enters your mind, say "Stop!" Then, by a conscious act of your will, replace that negative thought with a positive one. Quoting Bible verses and truths is the best way to achieve this.

Paul said in Romans 12:2, *"Do not conform any longer to the pattern of this world, but be transformed by the renewing of your mind. Then you will be able to test and approve what God's will is—his good, pleasing, and perfect will."*

Moment by moment we must *take captive every thought to*

make it obedient to Christ (II Corinthians 10:5). We cannot help the thoughts that come into our minds, but we can help what we do with those thoughts.

The most effective thought we can bring into our minds to replace a negative thought is a scripture verse or passage. Remember that Jesus Himself faced every temptation from Satan through quoting scripture.

Practice Replacement Therapy until it becomes a life habit. Do not become discouraged. Keep in mind that it takes only about thirty days to establish a new habit, but it takes three to six months to break an old one.

Start the Day with Happy Thoughts

The first two minutes of the day are among the most important. Our waking thoughts help set the tone for the rest of the day.

So often we fill our minds with anxious thoughts first thing in the morning. Our mental list of the things we feel we need to accomplish that day or worries from the previous day begin to flood our minds. Before the day barely has started we feel overwhelmed.

Our attitude for the rest of the day could be enhanced if we would take the first two minutes of the day to focus on God. Adoring Him, thanking Him, enjoying His presence will make even the cloudiest of days seem bright.

In turn if we practice the two-minute rule with others we can help them have a happier day. Greeting them warmly and letting them know they are valued first thing in the morning can change the direction of their day. A little goes a long way, and this little practice can have far-reaching effects.

Dealing With Depression

We cannot end this study regarding the destruction of happiness without addressing the issue of depression. Although there are many causes of depression, among those most overlooked are improper nutrition and poor lifestyle choices. Generally speaking, depression is the result of a chemical imbalance in the brain. This imbalance is often the result of poor eating habits, lack of rest, and stress.

Physical and emotional stresses cause our adrenal glands to pump an abundance of stress hormones into our blood streams.

Simultaneously, our seratonin levels are diminished. The result is a chemical imbalance that can lead to depression and anxiety. Following the principles of <u>The Creation Diet</u> will target many causes of depression and in many cases help to alleviate them. After only a few months on <u>The Creation Diet</u>, a lady in the first test group was able to stop taking the anti-depression medicine she had taken for seven years.

Considering the benefits of light and happiness to our physical well being, we should become more aware of seeking the Source of this light. As we develop our relationship with the Creator, we find that all areas of our lives—spirit, soul, and body—are affected positively.

SPIRITUAL APPLICATION

Before God introduced light into the world, darkness and emptiness characterized the heavens and earth. However, when God looked upon the world He saw not only what it was, but also what it would become.

The same is true for you. Perhaps you have seemingly hopeless areas in your life. A life without hope is full of darkness. God desires that you live not in darkness, but that you walk in His light.

With God, life is never hopeless. The Bible is full of glorious truths that confirm this. A few of these precious promises follow:

> *. . . With man it is impossible, but not with God: all things are possible with God* (Mark 10:27).

> *We have this hope as an anchor for the soul, firm and secure. . .* (Hebrews 6:19).

> *Be joyful in hope. . .* (Romans 12:12).

If we choose to live life on our own, without a relationship with the Creator, life becomes dark, for we have no Source of light: *Remember that at that time you were separate from Christ, excluded from the citizenship in Israel and foreigners to the covenants of the promise, without hope and without God in the world* (Ephesians 2:12).

51

Bring the dark, empty areas of your life to the Source of light! God already knows what beauty and purpose He has for those areas. Only He can take that which is void and without form and transform it into something beautiful and wonderful. He will do so each time we choose to obey His commandments and walk in His light, for He is not only the Creator—He is also the Re-Creator.

Dear God,

Today I bring You all the areas of my life that are dark and empty. For too long I have tried to fix them on my own. Please take my life and help it become what You intend it to be. I bring my life to Your light.

In Jesus' name I pray, Amen.

MEMORY VERSE(S) FOR CHAPTER ONE:
The Lord is my light and my salvation. . . (Psalm 27:1a).

ASSIGNMENT(S) FOR CHAPTER ONE:

1) **Focus on God** first thing in the morning, last thing at night, and throughout the day. Establish a time each day for prayer and Bible study and worship.

2) **Think happy thoughts.** Make a conscious effort to replace negative thoughts with positive ones—thought by thought.

DEVOTIONAL FOR CHAPTER ONE

Day One

Scripture Reading: Isaiah 55:1-13

Verse of the Day: *I am the light of the world. Whoever follows me will never walk in darkness, but will have the light of life* (John 8:12).

The *light of life. . .* what a beautiful phrase! There are few, if any of us, who would choose to walk in darkness when we could walk in light. Have you ever gotten out of bed in the night and groped through the darkness to keep from disturbing others who were asleep? What happened? Chances are you either stubbed your toe, or ran into something, or maybe both. Do you remember the relief you felt when you entered a room where you could turn on the light without awakening anyone?

David declares that his salvation comes from the Lord who is his light. Jesus affirms that <u>He</u> is that light. He also explains that He is the way, the truth, and the life. It is not possible to come to the Father except through Him (John 14:6).

This is the very core of the Christian faith. To come to the light of this truth is where salvation is found.

- Admit that you are a sinner.
- Confess your sinful condition and make the choice to accept God's provision for you.
- Believe that when Jesus died on the cross, He became the sacrifice for your sins. His blood covers your sinful condition, and you are made right with God.
- Pray the prayer of faith by which you acknowledge that you accept what God has done for you through the death of His Son.
- Surrender to Him by inviting Jesus to come into your heart and allow the Holy Spirit to take control of your life.

When you make this commitment, you step out of the darkness into the light. To paraphrase the apostle John, *Children, keep on walking!* (III John 1:4)

<u>Application</u>:
1) The most important question you ever will face is "Have you come to the Light of salvation?"
2) If so, when and how?
3) What was your life like before that decision?
4) How has your life changed since you accepted Jesus?

PRAY for God's light to shine on you and show you how to walk with Him.

DEVOTIONAL FOR CHAPTER ONE

Day Two

Scripture Reading: Acts 8:1-3; 9:1-18

Verse of the Day: *Arise, shine, for your light has come, and the glory of the Lord rises upon you* (Isaiah 60:1).

One can almost see Isaiah's face aglow as he declares the magnificent truth of the glory of God's light. George Friderick Handel majestically set this verse to music. While composing "The Messiah," Handel felt God's presence by his side. Later someone expressed to him that everyone admired his work. Handel responded that his desire was not that his listeners admire his work. Rather, he hoped his music would make them better people.

Only the glory of God's light can make us better people. Faye Burgess Abbas, a singer who is blind, has inspired thousands of people through her music. I first met Faye when she was a fifteen-year-old student at the school for the deaf and blind where I taught. She was led onto the stage during a concert to sing one song. That one song impacted my life in such a way that even now tears fill my eyes when I think of it.

She stood there in a flowing yellow gown as her high soprano voice pleaded, "Savior, Like a Shepherd Lead Us." Faye is beautiful, and the song is beautiful. However, that is not what impacted my life in such a way. Something else made that a memorable experience.

It was apparent through the way she sang that Faye knew the Shepherd personally. He had indeed led her from her physical darkness to His spiritual light. And, the glory of the Lord was risen upon her!

Application:
1) Do people see the glory of the Lord in your life?
2) How do you know?
3) What can you do to allow His glory to shine through you?
4) Are you willing to do it?

PRAY for your life to be so filled with the glory of God that it shines on those around you.

DEVOTIONAL FOR CHAPTER ONE

Day Three

Scripture Reading: Matthew 5:13-16

Verse of the Day: *You are the light of the world* (Matthew 5:14).

What an honor Jesus has given us with this statement! We are the light of the world. What a responsibility Jesus has given us with this statement! We are the light in a very dark world.

The same word for *light* is also used when Jesus proclaims that He is the light of the world. How can that be? Jesus explains that when we come to faith in Him, He lives in us and we live in Him (John 15:4). Therefore, we simply reflect the Light that is within us.

As you travel a dark road at night, you may notice the reflectors on the side of the road do not give their own light. They only glow when in the direct line of car lights, thus reflecting the headlights. The same is true of us. We are merely reflections of the Light of the world.

When leaving New York City via the Lincoln Tunnel at night, there is a breath-taking view of the city. The panorama of lights is spectacular to behold. One night, as my husband was driving out of the city, he looked back at the dazzling display of lights. Suddenly, he remembered the hurting people he had encountered as he walked down the streets of the city. God inspired him with the following song:

> *The lights of the city are so beautiful,*
> *but the darkness of the city is sad.*
> *For there are millions of faces*
> *crying out from different places,*
> *yearning to be glad.*
> *The Light of the city is our Jesus.*
> *He's the bright and shining star.*

He needs you and He needs me,
wherever we may be,
to share His light wherever we are.
Will you share His light wherever you are?

Application:
1) Is your life a daily reflector of His light?
2) Where is darkness in your personal world? In the world around you?
3) What steps will you take to keep your light shining brightly?

PRAY and ask God to use you to share light in a very dark world.

DEVOTIONAL FOR CHAPTER ONE

Day Four

Scripture Reading: Matthew 5:1-12

Verse of the Day: *Now that you know these things, you will be blessed if you do them* (John 13:17).

Have you ever noticed that in The Declaration of Independence, Thomas Jefferson does not list "happiness" as an inalienable right? He lists "the pursuit of happiness." Perhaps our wise forefather knew that people must pursue happiness to obtain it.

In today's scripture reading, Jesus shows us how to both pursue and obtain it. He has given us the perfect prescription for happiness in the Beatitudes. Even the word *blessed* actually means "happy." These verses indeed should be-our-attitudes.

Have a repentant heart.
Admit sorrow for your sins.
Pursue meekness.
Protect righteousness.
Initiate mercy.
Nurture a pure heart.
Exemplify peacemaking.
Suffer persecution for godly living.
Sing and praise when falsely accused for the kingdom's sake.

Are these the things we seek in our pursuit of happiness? They are the only ways we ever will find it. In our world today, we seem to have confused "happiness" with "pleasure." If we look at this prescription for happiness, many of the things on the list would not be considered pleasurable, would they?

An article in the Miami Herald expressed the same sentiment. The article stated that happiness is not a commodity, but a condition. It is not freedom from pain, but the ability to turn pain into power. It comes neither from owning, nor from the lack of owning possessions. It comes not from without, but from within the heart.

Jesus gave the blueprint for happiness: *You will be blessed if you do them* (John 13:17).

Application:
1) What does "happiness" mean to you?
2) What do you consider the happiest time of your life? What made it so?
3) Have you been taking Jesus' blueprint into account in your pursuit of happiness?

PRAY and ask God to help you distinguish the difference between happiness and pleasure in your walk with Him.

DEVOTIONAL FOR CHAPTER ONE

Day Five

Scripture Reading: Luke 10:30-37

Verse of the Day: . . . *but blessed is he who is kind to the needy* (Proverbs 14:21).

Happiness is a funny thing (pardon the pun). It seems that the best way to get it is to give it away. Have you ever noticed that when you make someone else happy, it makes you happy? Do you think possibly that is what God had in mind all along?

Someone wisely said that happiness cannot be given; it only can be exchanged. That is why Paulus could say, "What is done for another is done for oneself."

I read a story once about a king who suddenly became very ill. The physicians in his court tried every remedy they knew and nothing worked. In desperation they brought in the finest doctor in the land. Upon arriving at the castle and assessing the king's condition, the doctor gave the following prescription: find the happiest man in the kingdom and bring his shirt back to the castle. If the king wore the happy man's shirt, he would recover.

The search began. Squires and pages left the castle, scouring the land looking for the happiest man. Day after day they searched. Finally, they were led to the home of the happiest man in all the land. Eagerly they rushed inside to take his shirt, only to find he no longer had one. He already had given it away.

Do you want to be happy? Make someone else happy!

Application:
1) Recall a time when you know you did something that made another person happy.
2) How did that make you feel?
3) Recall a time when you know you did something that made another person unhappy.
4) How did that make you feel?
5) What can you learn from these experiences?

PRAY and ask God to give you the opportunity to make someone happy. Enjoy!

DEVOTIONAL FOR CHAPTER ONE

Day Six

Scripture Reading: Psalm 146:1-10

Verse of the Day: *I think myself happy, King Agrippa, because I shall answer for myself this day. . .* (Acts 26:2 KJV).

We are as happy as we *think* we are. When Paul said, *I think myself happy* he used a wonderful choice of words. We can either think ourselves happy, or think ourselves unhappy.

Only *we* can control the thoughts we dwell on daily. Our thoughts evoke the emotions that lead to our behaviors, which eventually become our habits. Elbert Hubbard is quoted as saying, "Happiness is a habit—cultivate it." Solomon said, *"For as a man thinketh in his heart, so is he"* (Proverbs 23:7 KJV).

How can we *think* ourselves *happy* in the midst of troubling circumstances? The answer lies in Psalm 146:5: *Blessed is he whose help is in the God of Jacob, whose hope is in the Lord his God.* What more could we ever need than the assurance of God's help no matter what we are facing? That is our hope. That is our happiness. Dwelling on God's love and seeking His will keeps our thoughts where they should be—on Him.

The story is told about two construction workers who sat down to eat lunch. One opened his lunch box and began eating. The other pulled a sandwich out of his lunch bag and began complaining. He grumbled because he had another bologna sandwich. For five straight days he had eaten a bologna sandwich. Now here was another one! His co-worker suggested he tell his wife that he was tired of bologna. He looked at his friend and replied, "My wife? I fix my own lunches."

We are the ones who put the bologna in our minds. We, like Paul, can change our thought patterns by "thinking ourselves happy."

Application:
1) If your happy thoughts were graded based on 100% as a perfect score, what would be your grade?
2) What steps do you need to take to cultivate the habit of happiness?

PRAY and thank God for all the things He has given to make you happy. Ask for forgiveness when you fail to appreciate them.

DEVOTIONAL FOR CHAPTER ONE

Day Seven

Scripture Reading: Revelation 21:1-27

Verse(s) of the Day: *The city does not need the sun or the moon to shine on it, for the glory of God gives it light, and the Lamb is its lamp* (Revelation 21:23).

He will wipe every tear from their eyes. There will be no more death or mourning or crying or pain, for the old order of things has passed away (Revelation 21:4).

God began creation with the words "*Let there be light. . .*" (Genesis 1:3). The Hebrew word for *light, (owr)* literally means "luminousness and happiness." Before God finished creating the world He bathed it in His light and happiness.

From our scripture reading we see that, at a future time, the world we know will no longer exist. New heavens and a new earth will replace the world we have known.

Throughout Revelation 21 we read that one distinguishing characteristic of this new world is light! John, the author of Revelation, explains that the New Jerusalem *shone with the glory of God, and its brilliance was like that of a very precious jewel, like a jasper, clear as crystal* (v.11). In this city there is no need for a sun or moon, . . .*for the glory of God gives it light, and the Lamb is its lamp* (v.23).

Another distinguishing characteristic of this new home is happiness! There will be no. . . *tears. . . death. . . mourning. . . crying. . . pain* (v.4) anymore! Can you imagine how wonderful that will be? The light and happiness, which God intended for His creations, finally will be a reality. The darkness and misery of sin no longer will steal the Creator's gifts from His creations. As the song says, "What a Wonderful World" it will be!

However, there is a sobering thought that brings me back to the reality of the world in which we live presently. The Bible is clear that the wonderful new world of light and happiness referred to in this scripture is prepared for those who choose to have a relationship with the Source of light— the Lamb (Revelation 21:24). On the contrary, *the. . . unbelieving do not share this promise* (v.8).

What are our purposes for being in this present world? They are to develop a personal relationship with the Creator and help lead others to the Source of light. The result will be light and happiness, here and hereafter, this world and the next! *Let there be light!* (Genesis 1:3)

Application:
1) Search your heart to see if you are prepared to walk in the New Jerusalem.
2) What are you doing to lead others from darkness and misery to light and happiness?

PRAY and ask the Creator to shine His light and happiness in and through you!

CHAPTER TWO

BIBLICAL APPLICATION

The Second Day of Creation

(Genesis 1:6-8)

6 And God said, "Let there be an expanse between the waters to separate water from water." 7 So God made the expanse and separated the water under the expanse from the water above it. And it was so. 8 God called the expanse "sky." And there was evening, and there was morning — the second day.

Again, let us remember the basic premise of <u>The Creation Diet</u>. Through the creation narrative, God gave the design of how to live healthy, happy lives. He revealed the pattern, sequentially listed in the order of importance, of what is necessary for our total well being. The second day of creation further confirms this pattern.

You may recall that in elementary school classes we learned the "Rule of Three" for health. Our books taught us that we can live only three minutes without air, three days without water, and three weeks without food. Although modern scientists and researchers have debated the time frames suggested here, all are in agreement with the order for survival.

God already had conveyed these facts through the creative activities of the second day. On day one when God began the creation process with the introduction of light (happiness), scripture implies that the newly created world existed in a shapeless, watery

63

form. On the second day God gave shape and form to the world.

God summoned the waters into separation when He spoke, "*Let there be an expanse between the waters to separate water from water.*"

I. AIR

The upper waters were called *sky*. The sky houses the atmosphere, or air. Throughout the Bible, the sky is referred to as the handiwork of God. In Psalm 19:1 the Psalmist powerfully wrote that *the heavens declare the glory of God; the skies proclaim the work of his hands.*

The Creator himself gave the sky its intended purpose. It was designed to divide the upper and lower waters (Genesis 1:6). Its function is simple, yet complex. The sky holds the atmosphere that surrounds the earth. This air supports all life, plant and animal, and keeps everything alive. Without the moisture in the air (drawn up into the sky when God separated the waters) plants would die. The water in the ground, absorbed by plants, would be evaporated through the plant leaves. Without atmospheric water showering back upon the ground, vegetation would die.

Likewise, if the air drawn into our lungs were not moist, then we would wither and die. We would breathe out the fluids in our tissues and be left dry and lifeless. God knew this, so He created a beautiful abode for the atmospheric vapor known as air.

Jesus recognized the importance of the atmosphere. In fact, He used it as an example of one of the most profound truths of all times. Jesus taught a Pharisee named Nicodemus that, . . . *the wind blows wherever it pleases. You hear its sound, but you cannot tell where it comes from or where it is going. So it is with everyone born of the Spirit* (John 3:8). He explained that the wind's activity is a mystery. We cannot see it visibly, but can hear it, experience its effects, and feel it.

The same is true of the Holy Spirit. We cannot see Him visibly, but we can hear Him, experience His effects, and we most definitely can feel the Holy Spirit. Amazingly, the same Greek word, *pneuma*, is used for both *wind* and *spirit*. This principle holds true for the Hebrew word *ruwach* that also means *wind* and *spirit*.

II. <u>WATER</u>

The second act of the second day involved the lower waters that were left on the earth (Genesis 1:7). Knowing that water is vital for the existence of plant and animal life, God left enough water on earth to fulfill its necessary functions. The cycle of evaporation and condensation helps to sustain life on earth.

Jesus understood the necessity of water. Have you ever thought about how much of Jesus' life and teachings relate to water? The first recorded appearance of His public ministry was at the Jordan River where His cousin, John, baptized Him. As He emerged from the water, God declared, *"This is my Son, whom I love; with him I am well pleased"* (Matthew 3:17).

Jesus called His first disciples, Andrew and Peter, while walking by the Sea of Galilee. He used the water of the sea to illustrate that by following Him, they would become more than fishermen. They would become fishers of men (Matthew 4:18-22).

His first miracle was performed at a wedding where He turned water into wine. This was done out of obedience to His mother who beckoned Him to save the banquet host from embarrassment (John 2:1-11).

Jesus taught Nicodemus that to have a relationship with God, a person must be born of the Spirit (spiritual birth) as well as born of water (physical birth) (John 3:5).

He encountered a Samaritan woman at Jacob's well and offered her Living Water that would quench her thirst forever (John 4:4-42).

Many of Jesus' teachings were delivered either on the shore of a lake, sea, or river, or from a boat in the water. Once, when Peter had been fishing unsuccessfully all night, Jesus asked him to push further into the water and let down his nets. Jesus rewarded Peter's obedience by giving him a catch so great it broke his nets and he had to call for help (Luke 5:1-11).

When a storm arose on the Sea of Galilee late one night, Jesus' frightened disciples awakened Him from a deep sleep on the boat. With the words, *"Quiet! Be still!"* Jesus stopped the winds and taught the disciples that He is more powerful than any storm they ever would encounter (Mark 4:35-41). Immediately afterwards, He healed a demon-possessed man by sending the torturing spirits into a heard of swine, causing them to drown in a lake (Mark 5:1-20).

As the disciples were battling for their lives on a stormy sea at night, Jesus walked across the water to save them (Matthew 14:24-36).

Once, when He and His disciples were required to pay taxes, Jesus taught them a lesson in faith. He asked Peter to cast a hook into the sea, and open the mouth of the first fish he caught. Inside the mouth of the fish was the money they needed for the taxes (Matthew 17:24-35).

On the final night of His life on earth, Jesus used water to teach the importance of humility through serving others. Before the Passover meal, He initiated the ceremonial washing of the hands. However, He not only observed the ritualistic cleansing, He carried it a step further by getting on His knees and washing the feet of each disciple (John 13:1-17).

Water, that precious life-giving substance, was important in the life of our Savior. His haunting words from the cross were, *I am thirsty* (John 19:28). In life and in death, Jesus recognized the importance of water.

I am thirsty. God knew that water was vital to our well being, and He provided it from the beginning of time.

NUTRITIONAL APPLICATION

I. AIR (OXYGEN)

Air is necessary for health and well being. Without the pressure from the air around us, our bodies literally would fall to pieces. Air nourishes our bodies. Air conveys, refracts, and decomposes light. Air transmits sound. Air carries toxins from the ground and scatters them in the wind. Literally every physical and chemical process is made possible by air. God knew this, thus He placed it in an order of priority in the week of creation.

The great poetess, Elizabeth Barrett Browning, once wrote, "He lives most life whoever breathes most air." How true that statement is! Air is composed of 20% oxygen, less than 1% carbon dioxide, and the rest nitrogen. Oxygen is vitally important to the body's health.

Dr. Otto Warburg, President of the Institute of Cell Physiology, states that increasing oxygen to the cells is essential for fighting disease and producing energy. Dr. Sheldon Hendler, author of <u>The Oxygen Breakthrough</u>, notes that the oxygen available to the body through deep breathing strengthens the immune system and actually can rid the body of chronic illnesses.

How Oxygen is Obtained

Approximately 90% of the oxygen used by the body is obtained through breathing. The other 10% comes from food. On the average, a man breathes between 12-14 times per minute and a woman between 14-15. That amounts to approximately 20,000 breaths per day.

Benefits of Oxygen

Oxygen's benefits to health are numerous. Our busy brains use oxygen quickly. Lack of oxygen for 4-5 minutes will cause permanent brain damage in most people.

- Sufficient oxygen to the brain increases mental concentration. I encouraged my students at a technical college where I taught to relax and breathe deeply before and during tests. Taking the time to do so clears the mind and enhances thinking. In the same way, the physical function of correct deep breathing helps one's emotions. When the body is under stress, stomach muscles tighten and breathing becomes shallow. Employing deep breathing techniques helps to reduce stress by getting more oxygen to the brain.
- As mentioned in the beginning chapter, energy is produced when carbohydrates and oxygen are burned. Therefore, oxygen is vital for energy production and endurance.
- Pain often can be reduced through conscious, deep breathing. Natural childbirth classes are examples of this benefit.
- In addition, 70% of the toxins in the body are discharged through breathing. Without proper breathing and expulsion of toxins, other systems responsible for toxin removal become overworked and weakened.
- Our muscular hearts require oxygen to stay healthy and well. The tiny structure in the brain, called the medulla, is responsible

for reading the amount of carbon dioxide (waste material) in the blood. When the ratio of oxygen to carbon dioxide becomes imbalanced, the heart works harder trying to oxygenate the blood. This results in increased blood pressure.

The profound relationship between a healthy heart and proper breathing merits an explanation of the anatomy and physiology involved in each system. The following summary is provided:

Respiratory System

When we breathe correctly, we inhale through the nose. Our nostrils are filled with tiny nose hairs that filter dust and debris. We also have a mucus blanket that lines our nostrils and runs down the trachea into the bronchi of the lungs. This mucus membrane helps trap infiltrates and is filled with white blood cells that attack germs. Therefore, as we inhale, the air is cleansed as it travels into the lungs. Since there is an "out" breath for every "in" breath, moisture from the out breath is deposited in the mucus blanket.

From the nostrils, air travels into a tube called the trachea. It then moves into smaller passageways, the bronchi and bronchioles. Finally, air reaches the tiny sacs named the alveoli. If it were possible to open and spread out all these tiny sacs, they would cover a basketball court. All day and night these little alveoli pass oxygen into the blood where it is taken to the heart and pumped throughout the body. The blood then brings carbon dioxide, a waste product, from the cells back to the alveoli where it is exhaled through the mouth.

Truly the human body is amazing. Each breath we take is a gift from God who shared His very own breath with us.

Circulatory System

We have over 96,000 miles of circulatory system in our bodies. The human heart, a muscle about the size of a man's fist, weighs a little more than one-half pound. All day long for a lifetime, this small muscle pumps 6 quarts of blood throughout the body every minute, averaging 70 beats each minute. That equals 4200 beats per hour, 100,800 beats per day. In a year's time, the heart pumps enough blood to fill between 97 to 200 tank cars with a holding capacity of 8,000 gallons each.

The heart has four chambers including two atria and two ventri-
cles. Through a system of arteries, veins, and capillaries the miracle
of a beating heart takes place. The right atrium receives "used"
blood from the body, then pushes that blood into the lower right
ventricle. From there it is sent up to the lungs where carbon dioxide
is exchanged for oxygen. The oxygenated blood descends to the left
atrium where it is sent down to the left ventricle and on throughout
the body. The cycle then begins again. Minute by minute our hearts
work harder than we can imagine to keep us alive.

Importance of Deep Breathing
It is very important to note that most blood flow occurs in the
bottom third of the lung. Therefore, deep breathing is crucial for
oxygenation of the blood.

The diaphragm is a thin sheet of strong fiber located between
the bottom of the lungs and the top of the abdomen. When we
breathe correctly, it flattens and expands. This enables breath to get
to the bottom of the lungs where the blood-flow occurs.

A direct correlation exists between shallow chest breathers and
heart trouble. In a Minneapolis hospital, 153 heart-attack patients
were examined. It was found that all 153 were shallow chest
breathers. In addition, 76% of them were found to inhale through
the mouth rather than through the nose.

How To Breathe Deeply
How can we make sure we are breathing correctly? Babies
know how! Watch as a baby breathes and you will notice two
things. First, the stomach muscles remain relaxed and as the baby
inhales, the belly becomes full and round. Second, the baby's spine
flexes a little with each breath.

The first step in improved breathing is to become conscious of
taking deep breaths.

1) Place your hand on the upper abdomen.
2) Slowly inhale through the nose.
3) Fill the chest to the point that the upper abdomen expands,
   causing your hand to move.
4) Slowly exhale through the mouth.

Become conscious of deep breathing as often as possible. The benefits are well worth the effort!

Exercise

If you simply are resting in bed, you inhale 8 quarts of air per minute. Sitting up doubles the intake to 16 quarts. An active sport, such as jogging, increases the inhalation amount to 50 quarts.

Exercise is crucial to health because it increases oxygen through breathing. In fact, increased oxygen is one major purpose of exercise since the most efficient exchange of oxygen and carbon dioxide takes place when deep breathing occurs. Moderate exercise produces an aerobic (with oxygen) state in the body, promoting the presence of stable oxygen molecules. However, over-exercising can produce an anaerobic (without oxygen) state that promotes the presence of unstable oxygen molecules, called free radicals, in the body.

Although there is not an element of the creation week that specifically corresponds to exercise, its importance is evident through the priority given to air in the narrative. The importance of some form of moderate exercise cannot be overstated!

Adam was created with a perfect body, yet even he was given a duty that would ensure he exercised moderately: *The Lord God took the man and put him in the Garden of Eden to work it and take care of it* (Genesis 2:15).

In addition, the fact that God gave the example of rest on the seventh day implies that man's consistent activity was foreseen. He knew that moderate exercise would provide the life-sustaining air He summoned into existence on the second day of creation.

Importance of Exercise

Not only does moderate exercise promote breathing and increase oxygen in-take, it also assists in the following:

- Increase of strength and endurance
- Reduction of tension and stress-related disorders
- Control of weight
- Purification of the blood
- Aid of digestion
- Improvement of the circulatory system

- Control of pain
- Improvement of posture

CHOICES THAT DIMINISH THE BENEFITS OF AIR

I cannot conclude this section regarding air without mentioning how we have allowed poor lifestyle choices to distort our use of God's priceless gift—air.

Lack of Exercise
Sedentary lifestyles rob us of the benefits of increased oxygen provided through moderate exercise.

Pollution
Everyday, toxic fumes are poured into the air through factories, engines, and modes of transportation. We have polluted this precious commodity so much that environmental factors are considered to be one of the major detriments to our health. Lead poisoning in the body occurs mainly from the air we breathe. It has been determined that 74% of children from heavily populated cities have dangerously high concentrations of lead in their bodies.

Smoking
Smoking produces a devastating effect upon the balance of the body. As nicotine enters the blood stream from the lungs and circulates throughout the body, it paralyzes the ganglia, or "switchboards," of the sympathetic nervous system. In addition, nicotine works against the adrenaline produced by the adrenal glands which slow down the normal movements of the intestines.

Nicotine causes blood pressure to rise. It contracts vessels in the skin giving it a pale appearance. It also causes the bile duct to contract, affecting the liver and the gall bladder.

Nicotine depletes vitamin C, and smoking has been proven to contribute to lung cancer.

God knew what we would need to stay healthy. One of the main provisions He gave for our health was pure, clean air. It is crucial that we make lifestyle choices that will preserve this important treasure.

II. <u>WATER</u>

Water—pure, clean, clear water is one of nature's most important nutrients. Nothing can take its place. It is the most common substance on earth. Almost three fourths of the earth's surface is covered with water.

The physical properties of water make it different from any other liquid. Water has the unusual quality of being lighter in its solid form than when it is liquid. God, in His infinite wisdom, knew that if water were the same as other liquids, ice would be heavier than liquid water. As such, it would sink to the bottom of lakes, rivers, or seas, piling up to the top and killing marine life.

Over sixty-five percent of the body is comprised of water. The blood is 90% water, muscle is 72% water, and the brain is 75% water. Bone is 30% water, and the skin is 71% water. Even fat is 15% water.

All cells, tissues, fluids, and secretions of the body contain high percentages of water. In fact, an average body contains 96 pints of water. Sixty-five of those pints are inside the body cells, and 36 pints are found in the bodily fluids—blood, digestive juices, and lymphatic fluids.

The processes of every system in the body involve water. Included in these processes are digestion, absorption, circulation, and elimination.

Water has the unique ability to store great amounts of heat. The internal daily processes of human beings create enough heat to raise their body temperatures by as much as 300°. However, the water stored in the body tissue helps to keep the temperature around 98.6° Farenheit.

Human tissues require at least 2½ quarts of water each day. Most people drink only about a quart or less per day.

God knows how vital water is to the health of the body. That is why He placed it in such a high priority in the creation week. Virtually every living cell, plant and animal, is dependent upon water for life.

Why is water so important to health and well being? Recall from the beginning chapter that *the life is in* the *blood* (Leviticus

17:11). Blood, which is predominantly water, transports nutrients to the cells of the body. It also carries poisons away from the cells to the proper systems of elimination. Therefore, like air, water is necessary for cell nourishment and toxin removal. It is impossible to have a healthy body without the proper amount of water.

If water stayed inside the body, it would not be necessary to drink it continuously. However, water constantly is being lost through the elimination processes of the kidneys, bladder, bowels, lungs, and skin. Through urine, feces, exhalation, and perspiration, between three quarts and a gallon of water is lost daily.

As far as scientists are able to determine, water as we know it has not been found on any other planet. We should treasure this natural, God-given resource for the value it imparts to our lives.

Benefits of Water

Besides carrying nutrients to our cells and transporting toxins away from them, water performs a host of other functions in the body as well.

- Water makes food digestion possible. However, it is best not to drink water with meals. Instead, drink it one-half hour before a meal. This enables the digestive juices and enzymes to work more efficiently without being diluted. Water is used most effectively when it is consumed first thing in the morning, between meals and snacks, and before going to bed.

- Water lubricates the joints and helps tone the muscles by preventing dehydration. Water helps prevent sagging skin, especially following weight loss. Shrinking cells are buoyed by water, and the skin is more resilient and clear. Also, water moisturizes the skin from within. Skin care specialists tell their clients that the single most important thing they can do for their skin is to drink water. In a nutrition class that I taught, one of the assignments was to increase the daily intake of water. I was amazed by how many class members reported improved skin conditions. One participant, who had convinced her husband to drink more water, marveled that he no longer used lip balm. He previously had an "addiction" to it, using it constantly. Perhaps this success can be attributed to the fact that the skin is 71% water.

- Water actually increases brain activity since the brain is 75% water. An insufficient amount of water will cause frequent headaches, dizziness, and even blurred vision.
- Water serves as a shock absorber inside the eyes and spinal cord.
- Water serves as a natural appetite suppressant by cleansing the taste buds from flavors that trigger cravings. Another way it acts as an appetite suppressant is by making the stomach feel full between meals. Hunger pangs have been compared to ocean waves. They begin, rise, reach a crest, then subside. The whole process of hunger only lasts about twenty minutes. Therefore, if water is taken when the wave begins, it will help to satisfy the urge to eat. (Also, remember when eating that it takes twenty minutes for the brain to realize that the appetite is satisfied. So, eat slowly, do not overeat, and keep in mind that it will take approximately twenty minutes to feel full.)
- In addition to suppressing the appetite, water also helps to metabolize fat in the body. The kidneys cannot function adequately without a sufficient amount of water, thus the liver has to assume part of their work. The liver, which functions to metabolize stored fat into energy, cannot do all of its work when it is doing part of the work of the kidneys. Therefore, the liver metabolizes less fat and more is stored in fat deposits within the body without sufficient water intake.
- Water prevents retention of water and solid waste material by keeping the body from going into a water deprivation mode. When the body does not get enough water, it begins to panic and fear dehydration. As a result, it retains the water it does have. When it receives enough water, it releases what is needed in the elimination process. Also, water prevents the retention of solid waste material by keeping the bowel moist and allowing normal bowel function. Without adequate water, the body siphons the liquid it needs from internal organs, especially the colon, and constipation results.

With all of these functions in mind, we should commit thankfully to consume this life-giving nutrient throughout the day, everyday! It has been said that eight glasses of water per day (8 ounces each) is an acceptable amount to maintain health. However, we are not limited to that amount. Ideally, we should drink eight ounces per twenty pounds of body weight each day. (To determine the number of 8 ounce glasses you should consume daily, simply divide your body weight by twenty.)

Remember to drink water throughout the day. Your kidneys are only a little larger than your ears, so you do not want to overload them by drinking too much at a time.

Since many water supplies are polluted, it is advisable to purchase water purified by reverse-osmosis, preferably ionized as well. Natural spring water is another wonderful choice but only if you are sure the source of the water is not contaminated. Research what is available in your area. Many companies will make home deliveries when water is purchased in certain quantities.

CHOICES THAT DIMINISH THE BENEFITS OF WATER

Our lifestyles have so distorted our thinking we often crave beverages other than the blessed water God has given us. The desire for the pure, clean nutrient provided through water has been replaced with the longing for coffee, tea, colas, processed juices with high sugar content, and alcohol. These substitutes throw the body chemistry out of balance, leading to disease and premature aging.

Caffeine

The caffeine found in coffee, tea, chocolate, and most soft drinks, is related chemically to uric acid. It stimulates the adrenal glands to produce hormones that, in turn, cause the liver to pour sugar into the blood stream. Over a period of time, this activity weakens the ability of the pancreas to utilize insulin that stabilizes the sugar level in the blood.

Caffeine stimulates the nerve cells, increases the pulse rate, and causes nervousness. It prompts the gastric glands to secrete more juices in the stomach, leading often to peptic ulcers and other irritations of the digestive tract. Kidney activity is increased causing large amounts of salts to be taken from the blood. Caffeine is also known to deplete Vitamin C and calcium in the body.

If one chooses to drink caffeine, certain teas (such as green tea) are less stressful to the body and also contain antioxidants. If the choice is made to stop drinking caffeine altogether, it is best to wean off by degrees rather than stopping abruptly. Abrupt cessation can cause strong detoxification symptoms. Simply decrease progressively the amount of caffeine consumed.

Soft Drinks

In addition to the caffeine in most soft drinks, various synthetic ingredients are added. Read the label on a soft drink and see if you recognize anything on the list. Soft drink companies use caramel coloring to give beverages their characteristic brown tint. The dye in them is suspected as a cancer-causing agent. Many soft drinks contain polyethylene glycol, an oil solvent also used in automobile antifreeze.

The fizz in a soft drink is caused by phosphoric acid. The phosphorous contained in phosphoric acid upsets homeostasis in the body, particularly the calcium-phosphorous ratio. Calcium is dependent upon phosphorous to function effectively, so an imbalance in levels of phosphorous in the body negatively affects the utilization of calcium. In a desperate attempt to acquire the usable calcium it needs, the body siphons calcium from bones, teeth, and elsewhere in the body. In addition, phosphoric acid weakens the activity of hydrochloric acid in the stomach, preventing adequate digestion and producing gaseous bloating in most people.

Many soft drinks come packaged in aluminum cans. Acid in the soft drink eats away the aluminum, which floats in the liquid. When consumed, this aluminum is very toxic in the body, particularly the brain.

Soft drinks contain high amounts of sodium, causing water retention in the body. After many years of ingesting soft drinks, the kidneys and bladder do not function adequately.

In addition to all of this, most soft drinks consist of nine teaspoons of sugar, the equivalent of 36 feet of sugar cane. In 1990, it was found that the average American drank 42 gallons of sodas (regular and diet), but only 41 gallons of water per year.

Sugary Fruit Juices

Many of the fruit juices on the shelves today have been processed with sugars and "enriched" with synthetic vitamins. Why does fruit juice which is naturally sweet need to be laden with corn syrup or other sweeteners?

We must beware of the heavy sugar content in fruit juices and not consume more than the body can utilize. Fruit juices should be diluted with pure water to cut down on the sugar content.

Alcohol

Alcohol is a narcotic (mind-altering drug) similar in chemical makeup to chloroform and ether. It is addictive and destructive. After an initial surge of stimulation, alcohol depresses the activity of the brain, causing reflexes to become distorted. It also interferes with the action of vitamins in the body, and hinders the digestion of vital foods by causing the red blood corpuscles to clump together in a condition known as agglutination. This thickens the blood and prevents oxygen from reaching cells connected to the tiny vessels called capillaries. Without oxygen provided by the blood, cells begin to die. Many cells are replaced within the body, but when brain cells die they never are replaced. In addition, alcohol is known to have a toxic effect on various organs of the body.

The Choice is Yours

In one corner we have water. All cells and systems of the body depend on it. It enters the body and is so pure it does not have to be changed in any way. It feeds the body and then carries away the waste. It helps keep the body in balance.

In the other corner we have coffee, tea, soft drinks, sugary juices, and alcohol. They poison every cell and system in the body. They have to be filtered by the body, but when broken down they have almost no nutritive value. They are known to cause imbalance in the body. They fill the body with toxins.

Which one do you choose as the champion?

SPIRITUAL APPLICATION

Nothing on earth can exist without air and water. They both are free. They are not expensive, yet they are priceless. They do not call attention to themselves, but they point to the Creator. They exist to benefit living things.

The same should be true of those of us who have come into a personal relationship with the Creator. The purpose of our lives should be to bring glory to the Creator and to benefit other people. We are told in John 15:8 that *this is to my Father's glory, that you bear much fruit, showing yourselves to be my disciples.*

What a valuable lesson we can learn from air and water! Like these two elements, we should allow our lives to be necessary, useful, and purposeful. Also, like them, our very existence should bring glory to our Creator and benefit others!

Dear Creator God,

Thank You for the air and water You have provided for us. You are so wise. You knew what we would need to experience health and well being, so long ago You created what we need. Please help us not only to use these resources wisely, but let us conserve them wisely.

In Jesus' name I pray, Amen.

MEMORY VERSE FOR CHAPTER TWO:
Jesus answered, "I tell you the truth, no one can enter the kingdom of God unless he is born of water and the Spirit" (John 3:5).

ASSIGNMENT(S) FOR CHAPTER TWO:

1) Perform at least **10 deep breathing exercises** a day. **Deep breathing**, preferably fresh air throughout the day, will help oxygenate the blood.

2) **Water** should be consumed throughout the day, with a goal of at least **8 ounces per 20 pounds of body weight.** (Divide your body weight by 20 to determine the number of 8 ounce glasses of water you should drink daily.)

DEVOTIONAL FOR CHAPTER TWO

Day One

Scripture Reading: Genesis 3:1-6; Matthew 4:1-11

Verse(s) of the Day: *As for you, you were dead in your transgressions and sins, in which you used to live when you followed the ways of this world and of the ruler of the kingdom of the air, the spirit who is now at work in those who are disobedient* (Ephesians 2:1,2).

Paul calls Satan *the ruler of the kingdom of the air.* Not only does this refer to his control of the fallen angels, but it also alludes to the influence of his evil spirits upon the world. Like air, they are invisible, yet they strive to draw people into worldly directions contrary to God's will.

Consider the ways Satan appears today through the air. Think of the temptations that come through television, radio, and the internet; all which depend on signals through the air. Notice the commercials that are prevalent each day. Do they advertise clean air, pure water, fresh vegetables, seeds (nuts, whole grains, legumes), fruits and wholesome meats? No! Most of the advertisements promote items that attack our health and well being.

Satan repeatedly uses the same tactics. Once we become aware of his tactics we can learn to avoid them. I John 2:16 warns that temptation comes through *the lust of the flesh, the lust of the eyes and the pride of life* (KJV). Satan used this pattern with Eve. In Genesis 3:6, Satan convinced Eve that the tree was *good for food* [lust of the flesh], *pleasing to the eye* [lust of the eyes], and *desirable for gaining wisdom* [pride of life].

Likewise, Satan used this same pattern when tempting Jesus. In Matthew 4:3, Satan instructed Jesus to "*tell these stones to become bread*" [lust of the flesh]; in Matthew 4:6 to "*throw yourself down*" from the temple to prove that the angels would catch Him [pride of life]; and in Matthew 4:8, Satan *showed him all the kingdoms of the world and their splendor* [lust of the eyes].

Whether or not we are able to control what comes our way in the form of temptation, we can control what we do about it. A country preacher warned his congregation that when he looks at his neighbor's watermelon patch, he cannot keep his mouth from watering, but he <u>can</u> <u>run</u>. And so can we!

<u>Application</u>:
1) Which tactic does Satan most often use to tempt you?
2) How can you combat his attacks in that area?

PRAY for God to strengthen you so that you will not fall prey to *the ruler of the kingdom of the air.*

<u>DEVOTIONAL FOR CHAPTER TWO</u>

<u>Day Two</u>

Scripture Reading: I Corinthians 9:24-27; Philippians 3:12-21

Verse of the Day: . . . *I do not run like a man running aimlessly. I do not fight like a man beating the air* (I Corinthians 9:26).

It was the bottom of the ninth inning. Excitement filled the air, for this was no ordinary game. The championship rested on the players' field performance. The team was losing by one run, bases were loaded, and they had two outs. Everyone there, fans and fellow teammates alike, considered Mark the star player, the ultimate chance for his team to win the championship. A thunderous roar came from the stands as Mark stepped up to bat at home plate. The crowd chanted, "Go Mark! Go Mark!" Scanning the spectators, he saw fans holding posters and signs throughout the stadium. Some read "MARK'S our man! We know he can!" Others exclaimed, "Get on your MARK! Get set! Win!" Then his eyes fell on one proclaiming, "We're #1! MARK it down!"

Mark felt more pressure than ever before in his life. As he bent to grab a handful of dirt to rub between his hands, he noticed anticipation on the faces of the players in the dugout. Tapping the bat on home plate a few times, he steadied his feet and crouched into his favorite batting stance.

The sound of the ball cracking the wood of the bat echoed through the ballpark. It was a foul to the left. "S-t-r-i-k-e one," yelled the umpire! With the second pitch, Mark slammed the ball, but it sped just behind first base. "S-t-r-i-k-e two," came the call.

Mark's hands began to sweat. The chanting of the crowd increased. Everyone, even the players in the dugout, rose to their feet. All eyes and all hopes were on Mark. He took a deep breath and settled back into his batting stance.

The pitcher threw the ball. For one millisecond, Mark's eyes veered to first base where he was preparing to run. He drew back the bat and with all the gusto he had, he swung as hard as he could. SWHOOSH! He had swung only at the air. Although it had been just one fraction of a second, Mark had taken his eyes off the ball as he glanced at first base.

Paul reminds us in today's scripture passage that if we do not keep our eyes on the prize, we are like a man who is fighting, but only beating the air. What is that prize? It is the heavenly crown promised to those who remain faithful to God throughout life. No reward on earth even can begin to compare to it!

Application:

1) Is there an area of your life where you feel you are *beating the air*?
2) What can you do to make your life more focused in that area?

PRAY for God to show you how to seek the prize of the crown that will last forever.

DEVOTIONAL FOR CHAPTER TWO

Day Three

Scripture Reading: I Corinthians 15:51-58; I Thessalonians 4:13-18

Verse(s) of the Day: *For the Lord himself shall descend from heaven...and the dead in Christ shall rise first. After that, we who are still alive and are left will be caught up together with them in* *the clouds to meet the Lord in the air. And so we will be with the Lord forever* (I Thessalonians 4:16,17).

Paul speaks here of what he calls a mystery because it is difficult to comprehend. Not everyone will die. At some point in the future, God will give the command, the archangel will shout, a trumpet will sound, and Jesus will descend from heaven into the air. From the air He will transport to heaven all those who have accepted Him as Savior and Lord. It will happen as quickly as the blinking of an eye. Our bodies will be changed from physical to spiritual bodies in preparation to enter His dwelling place. For those who are in Christ Jesus, the Bible calls this the *blessed hope* (Titus 2:13).

Jesus warned that we always must remain ready because it could happen at any minute. He said that not even the angels in heaven know the day nor hour, but the signs (fulfillment of Bible prophecies) will tell when the time is approaching.

With great emotion a friend shared the following dream: She was at an outdoor family gathering where her relatives were having a wonderful time. Suddenly she heard the sound of a trumpet. She could tell by the expressions on the faces of family members that only she and her children had heard it. Frantically, she ran from one to another screaming, "Did you hear that? Surely you heard that." The response from each one was, "Did we hear what?" As she and her small children began rising into the air, she saw the bewildered look on the faces of the relatives still standing on the ground. She and her children continued to rise, as those on the ground appeared smaller and smaller. Then the dream ended.

"Be Ready"
Be it morning, noon, or evening
Neither day nor hour we know
Only let us all be ready
When He comes with Him to go.
Ernest O. Sellers

Application:
1) Is the thought of the glorious appearing of Jesus a *blessed hope* to you? Why or why not?
2) If you knew that Jesus would return today, what preparations would you make for the event?
3) What keeps you from making those preparations now?

PRAY for God to reveal what you need to do to be ready for His return.

DEVOTIONAL CHAPTER TWO

Day Four

Scripture Reading: Exodus 13:17,18; 14:13-29

Verse of the Day: . . . *Do not be afraid. Stand firm and you will see the deliverance the Lord will bring you today.* . . (Exodus 14:13).

The book of Exodus specifically records that God did not lead the children of Israel in the way they expected. Instead of sending them along the shorter path, through Philistine country, He led them into what seemed like an impossible situation. The mass of people had followed Moses out of slavery in Egypt into the desert wilderness. Suddenly, everything seemed hopeless. There was a sea to the east, hills to the north and south, and an open valley to the west. Through this valley the sophisticated Egyptian army easily could overcome the unorganized crowd of sojourners.

They panicked. Sarcastically, they asked if Moses had brought them there to die as though he felt there were not enough graves in Egypt to bury them all. They begged to retreat and return to a life of bondage in Egypt. Moses' response was not what they had anticipated. *Stand firm.* When God leads you, even if it appears to be an impossible situation, *stand firm.* Moses proceeded to explain that they did not need to do anything except stand still. God would fight for them.

Then, in a miracle unparalleled in Old Testament history, God parted the Red Sea and allowed His children to pass over on dry land. Once they were safely across, He allowed the waters to flow back over the Egyptians and the entire army was drowned.

It is certain that when you follow God's leading, the enemy will pursue you. Satan will try to lure you into returning to a life of bondage. Yet those who have accepted Jesus Christ as Savior have been set free. They have walked across on dry land. They no longer have to fear the enemy. *Stand firm* and see God's deliverance.

In Ephesians 6:13, Paul tells us to put on the full armor of God so that we *may be able to withstand the evil day, and having done all to stand.* That relieves us of pressure. We do not have to fight the battle. It belongs to the Lord and it was won at Calvary!

Application:
1) What seemingly impossible situation are you facing right now?
2) Will you trust God to *part the waters* for you?
3) What fears do you personally need to let go of so you can *stand firm*?

PRAY for the faith to trust God in all circumstances. Ask for the courage to stand firm even when it looks as though the victory is impossible. Thank Him that He will not lead you where His grace cannot keep you.

DEVOTIONAL FOR CHAPTER TWO

Day Five

Scripture Reading: I Samuel 22:1,2; II Samuel 23:8-23

Verse of the Day: . . . *I was thirsty and you gave me something to drink. . .* (Matthew 25:35).

The setting of today's scripture reading takes place after King Saul had persecuted David for fourteen years. Saul was insanely jealous of David's popularity with the people of Israel. On many occasions Saul tried either to kill David, or have him killed. Saul exiled David from his beloved country, and he tried to turn the people against David. King Saul sought David on a daily basis (I Samuel 18-26).

It appeared that David had lost everything. Then, in the midst of his exile, David's father and brothers found him and helped him form a rag-tag army. In I Samuel 22:2 a description is given of the four hundred men who became David's soldiers. How would you like to be the leader of a stressed-out, debt-laden, discontented army such as David's? Yet he took what he had and made the best of the situation. David, whose name means "beloved," transformed this motley crew of soldiers.

Notice the description of those same men in II Samuel 23:8-23. They had become men who were mighty (v.8), leaders (v.8), committed and diligent (v.10), victorious defenders (v.12), loyal and courageous (v.16), famous (v.18), honorable (v.19), and valiant fighters (v.20). David accepted them as they were and he believed in them. He looked beyond what they were to what they could become.

The story in II Samuel 23:14-17 paints a beautiful picture of faithfulness, commitment, and bravery. David had been away from his hometown for some time and he longed to drink water from the well near the gate of Bethlehem. This craving came in the middle of a battle against some of his most fierce enemies, the Philistines. When three of his soldiers heard of his desire, they broke through enemy lines, went to Bethlehem, and brought water back to him. What love and loyalty they showed!

Can the same be said of our commitment? Our Commander, Jesus, takes us just as we are—stressed-out, debt-laden, discontented, or whatever our stance in life may be—and believes in us. He sees beyond what we are to what we can become. Are we willing to risk breaking through enemy lines to give a cup of cold water in His name?

Application:

1) Who is thirsty, in the spiritual sense, around you?
2) What would Jesus want you to do about it? Will you?

PRAY and thank God for choosing you to be one of His followers.

Ask Him to develop in you the same traits exemplified in the lives of David's mighty men.

DEVOTIONAL FOR CHAPTER TWO

Day Six

Scripture Reading: John 4:1-26; 39-42

Verse of the Day: . . . *Indeed, the water I give him will become in him a spring of water welling up to eternal life* (John 4:14).

One busy Saturday afternoon, I bought a piece of fried chicken at a market and devoured it in the car between errands. Then it happened. In my haste, I swallowed a rib bone of the chicken breast and it lodged in my esophagus. I quickly drove myself to the hospital emergency room where attendants performed the necessary x-rays and examinations. I called my husband and, as only a woman would do, asked him to vacuum the floor and clean the bathroom instead of coming to the hospital. (We were expecting guests for supper.)

I did not realize the seriousness of the situation. Before I knew what was happening, I was whisked to surgery after being given a medication to dry my mouth and throat. Later, after I was admitted to the hospital, the doctor warned I could not eat or drink anything until the next day. I begged the nurses for even a chip of ice to quench the thirst. They, of course, could not give me any liquids.

Jesus was tired from traveling so He sat beside Jacob's well. Along came a person who was the opposite gender (a woman), of another culture (a Samaritan), poor (she was drawing her own water), and an outcast (she was an adulteress). Jesus had mercy on her. Using the common substance of water as the basis for teaching, He explained to the Samaritan woman the way to eternal life. He revealed that it is a gift from God (v.10), obtained by asking for it from the Savior (v.10). He showed that the water He offered would well up into eternal life (v.14). In this one lesson, Jesus taught about the Father who provides the gift, the Son who gives it freely for the asking, and the Holy Spirit who lives eternally in each believer.

The next day when I awoke in the hospital, the nurses brought me a drink of water. However, as wonderful as it was, it in no way compared to the Living Water I received when I bowed on my knees as an eight-year-old child and drank from the well of eternal life—the same well from which the Samaritan woman drank many years before.

Application:
1) Have you quenched your thirst from the well of *Living Water?*
2) If not, will you accept that free gift from God right now?
3) If you have accepted God's free gift and the wellspring is in your heart, to whom do you need to offer the gift of *Living Water?*

PRAY and thank God for His free gift which leads to eternal life. Ask for the desire to thirst continually after righteousness in your life.

DEVOTIONAL FOR CHAPTER TWO

Day Seven

Scripture Reading: John 3: 1-21

Verse of the Day: . . . *I tell you the truth, no one can enter the kingdom of God unless he is born of water and the Spirit* (John 3:5).

Nicodemus, a religious leader, had a profound encounter with Jesus. Jesus' words not only challenged Nicodemus, they challenge people even today. What does it mean to be *born of water and of the Spirit?*

Nicodemus said the religious leaders (indicated by the *we* in verse 2) knew Jesus had come from God or He could not have performed His many miracles. Jesus, the master Teacher, responded by employing an important educational strategy. He piqued the student's curiosity.

Jesus told Nicodemus in verse 3 that unless a man is *born again* he cannot *see* (perceive) the kingdom of God. Nicodemus was shocked. He thought Jesus was saying that to see God's kingdom, a person would have to crawl back into his mother's womb to be born a second time. The strategy had worked. The student was hooked!

Jesus then proceeded with the lesson by explaining that a person must be *born of water and of the Spirit* or he cannot *enter* (v.5) the kingdom of God. "Seeing" the kingdom was important to Nicodemus, but "entering" was even more important.

Being a religious leader, Nicodemus was familiar with the *water*. The Jews had numerous rites of ceremonial washing and baptisms to purify themselves. One also was *born of water* when the sac of amniotic fluid broke during childbirth. But what did *born of the Spirit* mean? Nicodemus asked, *"How can these things be?"* (v.9)

Jesus, the Rabbi, then presented the heart of the lesson. The way to be *born again* is to be *born of the Spirit*. The way to be *born of the Spirit* is to believe in God's only begotten Son as the substitutionary sacrifice for the atonement of sin. Jesus' words in John 3:16 explained it all. *Believe* is much more than head knowledge. It is heart knowledge. The actual Greek word used is *pisteuo* meaning "to have faith in, to trust, to commit." Jesus taught Nicodemus that he *must* (v.7) be born again spiritually.

Air and water were the elements of creation associated with the second day. Water and Spirit are the elements of the re-creation associated with the second birth. The Greek word for *Spirit* is *pneuma,* which also means "a current of air." Air and water, water and Spirit (air)—that is certainly no coincidence!

Evidence confirms that the student learned the lesson. From John 7:50-52 we discover that Nicodemus defended Jesus before the chief priests and Pharisees, and John 19:39 teaches that Nicodemus brought spices to anoint Jesus' body for burial after the crucifixion. The Teacher was dying for you also to learn the lesson. Have you?

<u>Application</u>:
1) Have you had two "birthdays," physical and spiritual? If so, sing "Happy Birthday" to yourself twice! If not, today could be the day of salvation for you.

PRAY and thank God for allowing your birth and providing the way for spiritual rebirth.

CHAPTER THREE

BIBLICAL APPLICATION

The Third Day of Creation

(Genesis 1:9-13)

9 And God said, "Let the water under the sky be gathered to one place, and let dry ground appear." And it was so. 10 God called the dry ground "land," and the gathered waters he called "seas." And God saw that it was good.

11 Then God said, "Let the land produce vegetation: seed bearing plants and trees on the land that bear fruit with seed in it, according to their various kinds." And it was so. 12 The land produced vegetation: plants bearing seed according to their kinds and trees bearing fruit with seed in it according to their kinds. And God saw that it was good. 13 And there was evening, and there was morning—the third day.

PLANT LIFE

The new world, previously formless and empty, now acquired shape and fullness. By the command, *"Let the water under the sky be gathered to one place"* (Genesis 1:9), God established His intended designation for the water left on earth. With the words, *"and let dry land appear,"* the universal waters receded into oceans, lakes, and rivers.

This same command ordered the basic design of mountains,

hills, valleys, and shores. We as humans cannot imagine the power in the spoken Word of God. Standing at the edge of a vast ocean or climbing to the peak of a tall mountain puts this into perspective, realizing that God **spoke** this beauty and magnificence into existence.

The Psalmist captured this wonder when he wrote, *"But at your rebuke the waters fled, at the sound of your thunder they took to flight; they flowed over the mountains, they went down into the valleys, to the place you assigned for them. You set a boundary they cannot cross; never again will they cover the earth"* (Psalm 104:7-9).

God created this beautiful world with balance and purpose in mind. Even the geography of the earth is evidence of His orderliness.

One example of this is seen in the geographical formation of Jerusalem. In scripture, God referred to Jerusalem as the place that bears His name. A satellite view of this beautiful city shows that its valleys, the Hinnom, Tyropoeon (which is now filled with debris) and Kidron valleys, conjoin to form the Hebrew alphabet character *shin* (ש). In Hebrew thought, the *shin* written alone represents *Shaddai*, Almighty God. Geographically, the inflection point of the *shin* (ש) is the site of the former temple. God had ordained this as evidenced by His statement, *"But now I have chosen Jerusalem for my Name to be there. . . "* (II Chronicles 6:6), and Solomon's prayer at the dedication of the temple ". . . *this house I have built bears your Name"* (II Chronicles 6:33). God is amazingly accurate!

His intelligence is so far above human comprehension we cannot begin to fathom it. God, through the prophet Isaiah, expressed it beautifully when He said, *"As the heavens are higher than the earth, so are my ways higher than your ways and my thoughts than your thoughts"* (Isaiah 55:9).

God named the newly created dry ground *land* and the gathered waters *seas*. God now had made a dwelling place for life to exist. From the beginning, we have seen how God sequentially created things according to their importance for our health and well being. The world was no longer shapeless and empty, but was ready for its intended purpose. Even though it was still lifeless, God had equipped it to support life.

The first blessing of the third day occurred when God surveyed what had been created thus far and deemed that it was good. The

Creator was pleased!

God then called forth plant life on the earth. He called it forth in a planned order. There were three distinctive classes. First mentioned is **vegetation**, then **seed bearing plants**, and lastly **the fruit tree**.

The distinctions among the plant life seem to relate to the structure, the seed, and the importance to health. Structurally, in the first class, vegetation, the green blade is prominent; in the second, seed bearing plants, the stalk; and in the third, fruit, the woody texture of the tree.

In relation to the seed, vegetation has no conspicuous seed; seed bearing plants have noticeable seeds; and fruits have seeds enclosed within the fruit. Considering the importance to health, vegetables, then seeds or seed bearing plants (which include nuts, whole grains and legumes), and then fruits listed in categories sequentially relate to what is most healthful.

God decreed also that each of these would produce *according to their various kinds* (Genesis 1:12). He created the species of the world according to the characteristics that belonged to each of them. Although there may be variations within the species, their basic distinctive characteristics remain naturally to this day.

The waters were scattered into seas, lakes, and rivers. The land rose into mountains, hills, and valleys. Plant life proliferated through vegetation, seed-bearing plants, and fruit. Each was obedient to the Creator's summoning. Each was compliant with the task for which it had been created. Each is a clear example of unity in diversity.

God was pleased with what He had created on this day. In fact, He was so delighted He once again surveyed what had come into being and declared that it was *good*. This was the second time He affirmed the creative activities of the third day. The highest honor creation can receive is to be pleasing to the Creator!

NUTRITIONAL APPLICATION

The third day of creation pleased the Creator, for He knew that the newly created plant life would be imperative for the health of animals and man. Later, after the creation of Adam and Eve, God informed them that plants would be their food. *Then God said, "I give you every seed-bearing plant on the face of the earth and every tree that has fruit with seed in it. They will be yours for food"* (Genesis 1:29).

Genesis 1:11,12 mentions three categories of plant life—**vegetation**, **seeds** (including nuts, whole grains, and legumes), and **fruits**. The plants created on this day are the healthiest foods people can eat, because their natural forms contain nutrients necessary to keep the body perfectly balanced.

Vegetables, in their natural states, are vital to the nourishment of the body. Through their prolific varieties God provided many choices thus showing their importance to our health. Vegetables, primarily low glycemic, can be eaten in abundance, and the daily diet should include **at least 5-7 servings**.

Seeds (including most nuts, whole grains, and legumes) are excellent sources of fiber as well as protein and a host of nutrients. However, since many foods in this category promote acidity in the body by leaving an acid-ash after digestion, choices should be limited to **3-5 servings daily**. It is wise to choose ones that provide the highest amounts of fiber and lowest amounts of acidity.

Fruits have higher water content than any other foods. In their natural states, fruits not only provide the body with nutrients, they also act as cleansing agents.

Yet, fruits quickly convert to sugars which enter the blood stream. Adam and Eve were encouraged to eat an abundance of fruits. We must keep in mind, however, that they had perfect health and lived in a perfect environment. In today's society, as will be discussed later in this chapter, our bodies are bombarded with unnatural sugars. Therefore, it is best to limit fruits to **2-3 servings daily**. (Lifestyle changes that lead to eating less processed sugar will allow the consumption of more servings of fruit.)

The wonderful creations of the third day provide a variety of nutrients needed by the body. In His wisdom, God knew this, so He provided them for Adam, Eve, the animals, and us!

CLASSES OF NUTRIENTS PROVIDED BY PLANT LIFE

The body requires six main classes of nutrients—water, carbohydrates, fats, proteins, minerals, and vitamins. (Although other food factors, such as micronutrients, are important, they are not included in the six main classes of nutrients.) Miraculously, plant life created on the third day contains all six classes of nutrients.

The functions of these nutrients overlap to some degree, but they are designed for specific purposes. Many of the nutrients provide energy; others build, repair and maintain body tissue; and some regulate body processes.

The following is an examination of the six main categories of nutrients and their relation to plant life created on the third day.

I. <u>WATER</u>

Water's importance to the body was presented in the previous chapter. In addition, it is important to note that most plant life is comprised mainly of water. A watermelon is approximately 92% water, an ear of corn 70% water, and a tomato 90% water. Recall how your mouth fills with water upon biting into a juicy orange or stalk of celery.

We would benefit from becoming more conscious of the water within the unprocessed foods we eat. The closer we eat them to the way God created them, the more water they will contain. The majority of our diets should consist of these watery, life-giving plants created on the third day.

II. <u>CARBOHYDRATES</u>

Vegetables, seeds (including nuts, whole grains, and legumes), and fruits in their natural states are carbohydrates. The two types of carbohydrates are simple and complex, named according to the speed of digestion they initiate in the body. Most fruits and sugars are considered "simple" carbohydrates because they quickly convert into glucose and are pumped into the bloodstream. Most vegetables, seeds (including nuts, whole grains, and legumes), and a few fruits are considered "complex" carbohydrates because their molecular structure forces the body to work slowly while converting them into glucose.

The slow decomposition of complex carbohydrates produces heat in the body. The heat serves as a timed-release fuel that keeps metabolism working over a period of time. We acquire energy through the burning of carbohydrates, converted into glucose, and oxygen. God knew this and placed carbohydrates, especially vegetables, in a position of priority in the creation week.

Importance of Fiber

Carbohydrates, in their natural states, are comprised largely of fiber (cellulose). Although most fiber is not digested, it aids in the digestion of other foods. An adequate amount of fiber is necessary for proper digestion and elimination. Without it the body cannot expel waste from cells. Thus, toxins remain in the body and homeostasis cannot be achieved. The outcome is a poisoned body with a suppressed immune system.

The Standard American Diet (SAD) is high in fat and low in fiber. It is not unusual for a person who eats a low fiber diet to walk around with several pounds of fecal matter clogged in the intestine. To maintain proper elimination, approximately 30-35 grams of fiber are needed daily. The SAD is far below that level.

Importance of Chlorophyll

Scientists have discovered that the green-colored matter, chlorophyll, in plants is almost identical to the molecular structure of hemoglobin in human blood. Chlorophyll is responsible partially for the production of carbohydrates. As students in science class we learned of a process known as photosynthesis.

Photosynthesis produces carbohydrates when a plant containing chlorophyll receives carbon dioxide from the air, water from the soil, and light energy from the sun. Photosynthesis has been called the most important process in nature because it sustains all animals and humans. The chlorophyll that makes the production of carbohydrates possible also stimulates the growth of human tissue. In addition, it aids in the production of red blood cells and helps the body heal.

Acid-Alkaline Balance

Another crucial fact about the importance of carbohydrates is that many of them help create an alkaline condition in the body. After food is digested and the nutrients removed, an end product called "ash" is left in the tissues for some time. Ash can be either alkaline or acidic, depending upon the foods eaten.

Foods that produce an alkaline ash (above pH 7.0) in the body are called "base-forming" foods, and foods that produce acid ash (below pH 7.0) are called "acid-forming" foods. The ash left in our bodies has nothing to do with the taste of the food that produces it. Some of the best base-forming foods actually taste acidic, as in the case of certain fruits.

The opening chapter introduced the importance of keeping the base chemical balance at the proper pH level. As discussed in that chapter, on a scale of zero to fourteen (0-14), a balanced pH level is 7.0. However, cells function best and bacteria growth is limited when the body is slightly more alkaline. Research concludes that the best environment for a cell is between 7.2-7.365 pH.

Foods that leave an **alkaline ash** in the body are as follows:
- **Vegetables (most)**
- **Some unprocessed seeds (flax, pumpkin, squash, sunflower, and sprouted seeds)**
- **Almonds and chestnuts**
- **Fruits (other than cranberries and blueberries)**
- **Raw whey and raw cattle (goat and cow) milk**

Foods that leave an **acid ash** in the body are as follows:
- **Animal proteins**
- **Processed dairy products**
- **Most nuts (with the exception of almonds and chestnuts)**
- **Whole grains (except millet and quinoa)**
- **Legumes**
- **Vegetable oils**

The following substances leave no ash (because they supply no nutrients to be metabolized), but they have an **acidifying effect** on the body:
- **Alcohol**
- **Tobacco**
- **Drugs/medications**
- **Syrups**

- **Saturated fats**
- **Hydrogenated oils**
- **Sugars (processed)**
- **Artificial sweeteners**
- **Processed grains**
- **Table salt**
- **Drinks containing caffeine**

Once again, balance is the key. Many people go for weeks at a time eating only from the acid-forming foods. **The majority of the diet should come from alkaline-ash foods.**

However, some acid-forming foods, such as nuts, whole grains, and legumes are rich sources of fiber and nutrients. Therefore, they must be incorporated in the diet. Careful choices ensuring adequate fiber should be considered when selecting acid-ash foods.

Self-Checking Your pH

You can self-check your pH levels with either paper pH strips (litmus paper) or a pH electron meter. The pH paper strips are inexpensive and can be obtained from pharmacies, health food stores, or even educational stores. Most meters have to be purchased from health food stores or health catalogues.

Both methods can test your saliva and urine. Since different factors cause the saliva results to vary, urine testing is more accurate. Test the urine first thing in the morning. Evacuate the first drops of urine then catch some in a paper cup (or other container.) Place the pH strips in the cup.

The strips will change color to indicate the acid-alkaline base. A color chart accompanies the strips to help you translate the color into a number. Remember, the ideal number is 7.2-7.365. (If using a meter, follow the directions as printed.)

It is a good idea to check the pH at least weekly. Factors associated with daily living cause pH changes, so weekly testing gives a good overall assessment of the body's condition. Remember, disease is not likely to develop or grow in a balanced body!

CHOICES THAT DIMINISH THE BENEFTIS OF CARBOHYDRATES

Previous chapters presented how poor choices diminish the benefits of the blessings God intended through Light, Happiness, Air, and Water. Wrong choices also destroy the nutritional value of the creations of the third day. Often we desire and crave distortions of God's beautiful creations. We have become addicted to substitutes for wholesome foods, and we have unknowingly filled our bodies with toxins.

In our fast paced world, convenience replaces careful planning and preparation of meals. Our diets contain foods high in calories and fats, but low in nutritional value. When a young student was asked to name the basic food groups during a health class, she replied, "Wendy's, McDonald's, Hardee's, and Burger King."

Hosea 4:6 records God saying, *"My people are destroyed from lack of knowledge."* As we examine some of the choices that destroy the benefits of carbohydrates, it is my sincere desire that this section of Chapter Three will inspire commitment to healthy eating.

Processing

Unfortunately, most of the foods we buy in the grocery stores have been processed in some way. Even "fresh" fruits and vegetables in the produce section are grown with chemical fertilizers and sprayed with pesticides, fungicides, and herbicides. Before going to market, they are sprayed with preservatives to ensure that they look fresh for purchasing. The main purpose of modern processing, which began in the United States in the 1940's, is to give foods a longer shelf life. It seems that the longevity of the product has become more important than the health of the consumer.

The safest way to buy fruits and vegetables is to ask questions. It is advantageous to buy from local sources where you can inquire about the gardening process. As much as possible, avoid large grocery stores where the produce has been processed and imported from areas where you are not familiar with the farming procedures.

Refining Grains

Grains are full of wonderful nutrients and fiber. The term

"grains" refers to a variety of healthy plants. Some common grains are barley, brown rice, buckwheat, corn, millet, oats, quinoa, rye, spelt, wheat, and wild rice. A kernel of grain is comprised of the hull, bran, endosperm, and germ (also called embryo).

A Kernel of Grain

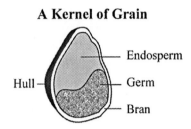

The hull (referred to in scripture as *the chaff*) has no nutritional value, so it is usually removed and burned. The purpose of the hull is to protect the interior of the kernel. The high fiber (cellulose) hull is not a nutrient, yet it helps give the kernel longer life. The bran consists of several layers, and its waxy outer coat further helps to protect the nutrients inside the kernel. Archeologists actually have found wheat in the tomb of the Pharaohs unspoiled after 4,000 years!

Progressing inwardly toward the center of the kernel, the layers begin to decrease in cellulose and increase in nutrients. The endosperm, the starchy portion of the grain, nourishes the germ. The starch is stored in tiny packets made of protein. These packets release the exact amount of nourishment at exactly the right time to keep the little germ fed until the leaves and roots of the plant begin the photosynthesis process. The kidney-shaped germ is a rich source of vitamins B and E, the two kinds of essential fatty acids (Linoleic and Linolenic acids), as well as protein. In Moses' song recorded in the King James Version of Deuteronomy 32:14, he refers to the *fat of kidneys of wheat* and the germ is kidney-shaped. Isn't God's Word amazingly accurate?

Food manufacturers found that when the bran and germ were removed from grain, the flour produced bread that would not spoil as quickly. Thus began the process of "refining" grain. "Refining" actually means "removal of impurities." How absurd that man calls the most nutritious part of the grain "impurities!" By removing the bran and germ from grains, manufacturers also discarded at least twenty-two vitamins and minerals. Then they began bleaching the flour to make it white, rather than the healthful light brown color it is naturally. Surely it breaks God's heart to see what we have done to His wonderful creations!

Harmful Effects of Processed Grain

Processed flour greatly endangers our health, for it causes a lack of balance in the body. The body is not equipped to handle man-made substances. Therefore processed flour becomes toxic and fosters a variety of diseases and illnesses. Unfortunately, bread is not the only product affected by this bleached, toxic substance. Pastas and pastries are affected, too. A careful consumer seeks unrefined sources of grain products, available in some grocery stores, health food stores, or through mail order companies.

Food Additives

The preservative chemicals added in processing are dangerous to the body. Scientific studies conducted shortly after grain refinement began showed significant deficiencies in vitamins B-1, B-2, B-3, and iron in the American diet. As a result, The Enrichment Act of 1948 forced food processors to add these four nutrients to processed flour. Thus, lifeless, processed grain now became "enriched" with man-made, synthetic nutrients created from a petroleum base.

In the name of progress various types of additives have been incorporated into the processing of foods. On the average, an American ingests more than a gallon of synthetic chemicals and additives, coloring agents, pesticides, and preservatives annually. Why do food companies add these harmful agents to our foods? There are several reasons.

Besides prolonging shelf life, manufacturers attempt to make foods more appealing to the sight and taste. For example, a hot dog wiener is actually gray in color, rather than red. The "nutrients" added by food producers are usually synthetic and unable to be used by the body.

In addition, chemicals are added in the processing to help emulsify, stabilize, and thicken the food. Other additives are used to leaven the food, to keep it from caking, or to give moisture. Some additives are used to try to maintain pH control.

Our bodies cannot easily digest all these chemicals that put particular strain on the liver as it tries to assimilate them. Checking labels is necessary in attempting to find foods as close to their natural states as possible. Man-made "progress" has actually endangered our lives.

Refined Sugar

Of all the toxins added to our foods today, refined sugar is one of the most widely used, as well as one of the most dangerous. It would be difficult, if not impossible, to enumerate adequately sugar's harmful effects on the body.

Actually, refined sugar could be considered a drug rather than a food. A *drug* is defined as any substance that produces a chemical change in the body and is addictive. Processed sugar is unnatural and it causes dependency. In its refined state, sugar is 99.4 to 99.7 percent empty calories. A simple carbohydrate, sugar contains no fat, no protein, no vitamins, and no minerals. Nothing in refined sugar is beneficial to the body. In fact, it is detrimental, and a host of degenerative diseases can be traced to the ingestion of sugar.

Sugar Consumption

Sugar was once a luxury item. In colonial America, it cost $2.40 per pound, and a cube of sugar in a Christmas stocking was considered a rare treat. When a large-scale method of granulating sugar was developed in 1795, Louisiana farmers began growing sugar cane as a major crop. As sugar prices decreased, sugar consumption increased.

A century ago, the average American consumed only ten (10) pounds of sugar a year. By 1958 the per capita consumption increased to one hundred-twenty (120) pounds and by 1994 it had increased to one hundred forty-nine (149) pounds. Recent statistics estimate that the average American consumes up to one hundred-sixty (160) pounds of sugar annually or over thirteen pounds of refined sugar a month!

Names of Refined Sugars

The refining process takes sugar beets, sugar cane, and corn that are full of vitamins, minerals, and fiber and strips them of their nutrients. Until the 1970's most processed sugar came from sugar beets and/or sugar cane, and was called sucrose, or table sugar. In the 1970's, manufacturers discovered that sugar from corn was less expensive to process, so corn sweeteners became the most popular way to refine sugar.

Since most processed foods contain some type of sweetener, it is important to know the names of the ingredients found on the labels. The presence of any of the following means that sweeteners have been added to foods:

- **glucose** (the type of sugar found in the blood, derived from food, and used by the body for heat and energy)
- **dextrose** (another name for sugar)
- **fructose** (found in fruits, juices, and honey)
- **levulose** (found in fruits)
- **invert sugar** (combination of sugars found in fruits)
- **galatose** and **lactose** (found in milk)
- **sucrose** (refined white sugar)
- **brown sugar** (refined sugar covered with a film of dark syrup)
- **molasses** (thick syrup separated when raw sugar is processed)
- **sorghum** (syrup from the juice of sorghum grain)
- **maple sugar** (syrup from the sap of the sugar maple tree)
- **maltose** and **dextrin** (sugars from starch)
- **mannitol, sorbitol,** and **xylotol** (sugar alcohols)
- **corn sugar** (sugar from breakdown of cornstarch)
- **"HFCS" high fructose corn syrup** (sugar from breakdown of cornstarch)
- **honey** (thick liquid produced by bees collecting nectar from flowers)

Hidden Sugars in Foods

Often we are not aware of the sugar hidden in many foods. One of the most difficult parts of controlling our sugar intake is finding which foods contain sugar. The following are examples of hidden sugar in foods:

- To improve the flavor and color of cured meats, many meat packers feed sugar to animals prior to their slaughter.

- Many fast-food restaurants add sugar to hamburgers to reduce shrinkage and inject chicken with honey to enhance flavor.
- Processed luncheon meats, bacon, and canned meats contain sugar.
- Syrup in canned fruits often contains sugar.
- Sugar is found in bouillon cubes, dry roasted nuts, peanut butter, many dried cereals, ketchup, and even some types of salt.
- The breading on most prepared foods contains sugar.

Our bodies need only two teaspoons of blood sugar (glucose) at any given time in order to function properly. Even if we never ate refined sugar we easily would acquire this amount through the digestion of carbohydrates, proteins, and fats. Approximately 10% of the fats we eat, 57% of the proteins, and 100% of the carbohydrates are capable of being turned into sugar by the body.

Therefore, every extra teaspoon of refined sugar we ingest works to disrupt the homeostasis of the body. For example, the body is able to handle only the equivalent sugar of one serving (1/2 cup) of fresh apples at a time. Some fruit juices contain as much sugar as the equivalent of four to six servings. The average candy bar has the sugar content of **at least** four servings of apples. **Even as little as two extra teaspoons of refined sugar can put the body into an emergency mode.** From this we can see how carelessly we treat the balance of our bodies when we abuse it with sugar day after day.

Harmful Effects of Refined Sugar

The ingestion of sugar upsets virtually every operation of the body. A chain reaction occurs in the body when too much sugar is consumed. The homeostasis of the body is affected, and the minerals of the body become deficient. Enzymes are dependent upon minerals in order to function correctly, so they are not able to adequately digest food. Particles of undigested food flow into the bloodstream, and the cells are unable to receive the nutrients they need from undigested food particles.

As a result, the immune system tries to rid the body of these undigested food particles. With time, this process exhausts and suppresses the immune system and the body becomes susceptible to degenerative diseases and conditions.

Diseases and Conditions Associated With Sugar

The following conditions and diseases are associated with the ingestion of sugar:

- Mental conditions such as hyperactivity, anxiety, irritability, drowsiness, lack of concentration
- Weakened immune system
- Kidney damage
- Elevated levels of triglycerides, cholesterol, and blood pressure
- Ischemic heart disease, cardiovascular disease, and arterosclerosis
- Obesity
- Tooth decay and gum disease
- Aging process and wrinkles
- Eczema
- Weakened eyesight, cataracts, and near-sightedness
- Mineral deficiencies
- Increased risk of certain types of cancers
- Arthritis
- Asthma and emphysema
- Formation of gallstones and kidney stones
- Increased size of the kidneys and liver
- Varicose Veins
- Hemorrhoids
- Peptic ulcers
- Osteoporosis
- Headaches, including migraines
- Hypoglycemia (low blood sugar)
- Hyperglycemia (high blood sugar resulting in diabetes)

Artificial Sweeteners

While attempting to avoid sugar, many people have added artificial sweeteners to their diets. There seems to be a false belief that artificial sweeteners are the lesser of two evils. Artificial sweeteners are exactly what the name implies, "artificial." They are man-made chemicals with no nutritive value. The human digestive tract is the same as from the dawn of creation, so it does not have the digestive enzymes necessary to handle man-made substances.

Types of Artificial Sweeteners

The two types of the most commonly used artificial sweeteners are saccharin and aspartame.

Saccharin is a coal-tar crystalline product whose label warns that its use may cause cancer. This artificial sweetener is found in Sweet'N Low, and Sugar Twin®.

Aspartame is a synthetic substance consisting of phenylalanine, aspartic acid, and methanol (wood alcohol, a poisonous substance). When aspartame is ingested, these elements are released into the bloodstream. Aspartame, two hundred (200) times sweeter than sugar, is found in NutraSweet ™ and Equal ™.

Splenda® is another popular artificial sweetener. Even though it is made from sugar, it has been converted into a synthetic substance by using chlorine atoms. Once again, it is "artificial" and unable to be used by the body.

Effects of Artificial Sweeteners

Some of the following effects are linked to the use of artificial sweeteners:

- Dizziness and loss of equilibrium
- Eye hemorrhages and tunnel vision
- Buzzing in the ears
- Muscle aches
- Numbness in the arms and/or legs
- Inflammation of the pancreas
- High blood pressure
- Hives
- Attention Deficit Disorder
- Memory loss
- Headaches (I personally found that migraines were linked to aspartame.)

What about my "Sweet Tooth?"

God wants us to enjoy life and the wonderful foods He created for us. The Bible presents "sweetness" in a positive way. However, that "sweetness" is associated with moderate amounts of naturally occurring substances, especially honey.

Throughout the Old Testament God refers to the Promised Land as a *land flowing with milk and honey*. In fact, the land is referred to in this way in Exodus, Leviticus, Numbers, Deuteronomy, Joshua, and Jeremiah.

The manna God sent from heaven to feed the children of Israel in the wilderness was said to taste like *wafers made with honey* (Exodus 16:31).

David refers to the ordinances of God as being *sweeter than honey. . .from the comb* (Psalm 19:10).

Solomon makes a positive reference to honey when he wrote, *"Eat honey, my son, for it is good; honey from the comb is sweet to your taste"* (Proverbs 24:13). In the next verse, Solomon compares the sweetness of honey with the fulfillment that comes from gaining wisdom.

King Solomon says also, *"Pleasant words are a honeycomb, sweet to the soul and healing to the bones"* (Proverbs 16:24).

When Isaiah foretold the coming Messiah, he uttered the immortal words, *"Therefore the Lord himself will give you a sign: The virgin will be with child and will give birth to a son, and will call him Immanuel. He will eat curds and honey when he knows enough to reject the wrong and choose the right"* (Isaiah 7:14,15).

This prophecy was fulfilled. Jesus appeared to His disciples after the resurrection, *and they gave him a piece of a broiled fish, and of an honeycomb. And he took it, and did eat before them* (Luke 24:42,43 KJV).

Honey is superior to refined sugar in several ways. Researchers have found 165 ingredients in honey including enzymes, minerals (two forms of calcium), amino acids (at least eighteen), and vitamins. Honey also contains natural antibiotic properties. Raw or unheated honey in its comb is best since heating destroys many of the healthful properties of honey.

The key seems to be moderate amounts of honey. Solomon warned, *"If you find honey, eat just enough—too much of it, and you will vomit"* (Proverbs 25:16). He further alerted that, *"it is not good to eat too much honey"* (Proverbs 25:27).

A word of caution: honey has been known to upset the digestive tracts of infants and small children, so it should not be given to a child under the age of one.

Other Sweeteners

Several other sweeteners are mentioned in the Bible. Freshly squeezed juices, dates, and even unprocessed sugar cane are referred to in scripture.

The herb, stevia, can be used as a sweetener and does not harmfully affect blood sugar levels as do other types of sweeteners. Due to its very sweet taste, only a small amount is needed to sweeten foods or drinks.

Learning to cook with natural rather than processed sweeteners is worth the effort in terms of benefit to the body. Many wonderful cookbooks are available with delicious recipes made from natural sweeteners.

III. FATS

Fats have received a bad name in our society because most people consume the wrong kinds of fats. It is true that God warned, *". . . Do not eat any of the fat of cattle, sheep or goats"* (Leviticus 7:23). However, the Bible also says, *"In this mountain shall the Lord of hosts make unto all people a feast of fat things"* (Isaiah 25:6 KJV). How could the Bible record in one place not to eat fat and in another to feast on it? The answer is found in the difference between what could be termed "bad fat" and "good fat."

The Hebrew word in Leviticus 7:23 is *cheleb*, meaning "to be fat; fat; the choicest part; grease, marrow." This verse is referring to "bad fat."

However, Isaiah 25:6 refers to "good fat." The Hebrew word for *fat* in this verse is *shemen*, meaning "grease, especially liquid (as from the olive)."

Amazingly, God showed through biblical Hebrew thousands of years ago that there is a difference between bad and good fats. According to scripture, the fat in most animal meat is "bad fat," and plant-based fats are "good fats."

Bad fats (saturated), coming from the fat of most animals, lead to a host of unhealthy conditions in the body. Good fats (unsaturated and monounsaturated), derived from plant sources, are beneficial to health because they perform a variety of functions in the body, including generation of energy.

Two Types of Good Fats

The body needs two types of good fats. The first type is the essential fatty acids (EFAs), which *are not* produced by the body. The other is the nonessential fatty acids, which *are* manufactured by the body.

Essential Fatty Acids

The two kinds of essential fatty acids are Linoleic Acid (LA) and Linolenic Acid (LNA). Both of these must come from the foods we eat. A good way to remember this is "it is **essential** that our diets include them."

Linoleic Acid (LA) (Omega-6 Fatty Acids)

Some of the main sources of Linoleic Acid include whole grains and most vegetable seed oils, such as sunflower and safflower. Also, olive oil, which is monounsaturated, is a healthy oil. The best choice is cold-pressed extra virgin olive oil bottled in dark glass.

Linolenic Acid (LNA) (Omega-3 Fatty Acids)

Food sources of Linolenic Acid include fish oils (especially from cold-water fish), marine plants, flax seeds and green leafy vegetables. Many of these are available in supplemental form for those who do not obtain them adequately through foods.

Eggs high in Omega-3 are available. They are produced through feeding flax seed and/or marine plants to chickens. As a result, the eggs contain Omega-3 fatty acids.

Important Functions of Essential Fatty Acids

Essential fatty acids help to assimilate fat-soluble vitamins; attract oxygen into the body; hold oxygen in the cell membranes (which keeps bacteria and viruses from growing); hold protein in cell membranes; promote gland secretions; metabolize foods; and carry nutrients into and out of cells. Since vegetables are among the most powerful sources of essential fatty acids, it is evident that the creations of the third day are vital to our health and well being.

Nonessential Fatty Acids

The body produces nonessential fatty acids. A way to remember this is "it is **not essential** to obtain them from our diets." Even though Omega-9 fatty acids are produced to some degree by the body, healthy foods are needed for fuel so the body can produce them adequately.

CHOICES THAT DIMINISH THE BENEFITS OF FATS

Saturated Fats

Fats and oils are made up of a combination of fatty acids. "Saturated fat" refers to the portion of saturated fatty acids in the fat. Saturated fats are found in animal products such as meat, dairy products, and eggs. Palm and coconut oils also are high in saturated fats. Too much saturated fat impedes or blocks the function of essential fatty acids in the body. The Standard American Diet (SAD) now consists of forty to fifty five percent (40-55%) saturated fat. This greatly contributes to the predominant fatal diseases in America, including coronary heart disease, strokes, and cancer.

Hydrogenated Oils

Once again man has taken something necessary for health and turned it into a health hazard. Essential fatty acids, not produced by the body, must be included in our diets. Food companies have taken healthful, unsaturated (polyunsaturated and monounsaturated) oils and hardened them through the process of hydrogenation.

Hydrogenation forces hydrogen molecules into the structure of vegetable oils at two hundred fifty degrees (250°) or more. From this process new fats, called trans-fats, are produced. The body does not know how to respond to trans-fats because they are man-made. We do not have the digestive enzymes necessary to process man-made substances. Through hydrogenation, healthful vegetable oils no longer remain unsaturated but are transformed into solid or semi-solid saturated substances similar to plastic. These transformed oils block the activity of essential fatty acids in the body.

Hydrogenated Products

Hydrogenated oils, including margarine and shortening, are found in a variety of foods on the grocery shelf. Since the body cannot utilize these plastic-like substances, they continue to collect in the veins and arteries contributing to a host of cardiovascular diseases. Margarine is so foreign to the body it has been estimated that one tablespoon can remain in the body for up to thirty-seven (37) days. Butter, in limited amounts, is more healthful to the body than margarine, because unprocessed butter is a natural substance.

Daily Consumption of Fat in the Diet

We should try to keep our consumption of fat to no more than twenty-five to thirty grams (25-30g) per day primarily from the unsaturated (polyunsaturated and monounsaturated) group. Some nutritionists advocate even less, suggesting an intake of fifteen to twenty grams (15-20g) daily.

Effects of Too Much Unhealthy Fat in the Body

The following is a summary of the negative effects of too much unhealthy fat in the body:

- Causes obesity (Remember: "Bad" fat is stored as fat in the body)
- Suppresses metabolism
- Raises cholesterol and triglyceride levels
- Lowers energy level
- Promotes cardiovascular disease
- Promotes cancer, diabetes, and other degenerative diseases

Remember: The vegetables, seeds (including nuts, whole grains and legumes), and fruits created on the third day contain very little fat and no cholesterol!

IV. <u>PROTEINS</u>

Proteins are the building blocks of our bodies. They are used constantly to rebuild our cells. If there is a shortage of complex carbohydrates or essential fats they can be used for energy. Proteins are comprised of amino acids. Twenty two (22) amino acids exist in all, nine (9) of which are essential to obtain from the diet since they are not manufactured by the body. A food that contains all nine amino acids is known as a "complete" protein.

Plant Sources of Protein

For many years it was believed that meat and animal products were the best sources of protein. Research now proves that edible plants, in their natural states, contain all 22 amino acids. Although the necessary quantity is not found in any one plant, eating a variety of vegetables, seeds (including nuts, whole grains, and legumes), and fruits helps provide a good balance of the protein that is needed by the body. The true standard of protein is its quality, and plant protein is of very high quality.

In addition, protein from plant sources is found to be easy to digest and assimilate in the body. Scripture tells of Daniel and three friends who refused to eat the rich diet of the king while in exile. They ate only vegetables and drank water. At the end of ten days their strength and health amazed the pagan king: *In every matter of wisdom and understanding about which the king questioned them, he found them ten times better than all the magicians and enchanters in his whole kingdom* (Daniel 1:20).

CHOICES THAT DIMINISH THE BENEFITS OF PROTEIN

As previously discussed in this chapter, we destroy the nutrients in the fresh, pure, raw plants God has given us for protein. We also are guilty of diminishing the nutrients found in the animal protein we consume. This will be presented in detail in later chapters when the creations of the fifth and sixth days are presented.

V. MINERALS

Important Functions of Minerals

Minerals are necessary for every chemical activity in the body. They give rigidity to the hard tissues of the body such as the teeth and bones, help maintain the pH balance of the blood, and transmit nerve impulses throughout the body. Minerals assist digestion and work synergistically with vitamins. Thus, they are predominant because all nutrients are dependent upon minerals for their activities.

There are eighty-four (84) known minerals and seventeen (17) are essential for human nutrition. Minerals work only in relation to each other, so if one mineral is deficient it affects the function of the others. The entire body can be thrown out of balance when there is a mineral deficiency.

Plant Sources of Minerals

Human beings were created from the *dust of the ground* (Genesis 2:7). All the materials in the composition of humans are found in the soil of the earth, including minerals. The body is not able to manufacture minerals from other substances, so it must receive them directly, or indirectly, from the soil. Since plants draw their nutrients from the soil, eating vegetables, seeds (including nuts, whole grains and legumes), and fruits allows us to ingest the minerals found in them. The importance of minerals to the chemical balance of the body cannot be overstated.

<u>CHOICES THAT DIMINISH THE BENEFITS OF MINERALS</u>

Minerals are not produced by the body and must be supplied through plant life. Plants derive their mineral content from soil, so the nutritive condition of the soil is crucial. Ideally, the topsoil in which plants grow is moist, dark, and filled with nutrients. The mineral-rich soil transmits the nutrients to the plants, which in turn transmit the nutrients to those who ingest them.

However, an alarming occurrence is happening worldwide. Due to soil erosion and degradation, the mineral content of soil is depleting rapidly. When America was colonized, approximately twenty-one (21) inches of topsoil covered the farmlands. Now, a little over two hundred years later, we have lost an estimated seventy-five percent (75%) of this vital resource and are presently down to about six (6) inches of topsoil. The soil that is left has become dry, lifeless, and depleted of nutrients.

Chemical substances added to enrich soil in no way compare to minerals that are present naturally when ecological farming methods are used. Sadly, one explanation for mineral depletion is that the soil of the land is not given a chance to rest and is "exhausted" from raising feed for animals to support our meat-based, SAD diets.

VI. <u>VITAMINS</u>

The word "vitamin" was coined while Caismir Fund was seeking the cause of the vitamin-deficient disease, beriberi. Unlike proteins, vitamins are not building blocks. Unlike carbohydrates and fats, they do not produce energy. However, they act as connectors that cause organic functions to take place in our bodies.

Two Kinds of Vitamins

Thirteen (13) vitamins are needed by the body daily. Two kinds of vitamins, fat soluble and water soluble, have been identified. Fat-soluble vitamins (A,D,E,K) can be dissolved only when fat is present. Without the presence of fat, they cannot be broken down and assimilated by the body. An accumulation of these vitamins can cause a toxic condition to occur. Water-soluble vitamins (C and the eight B complex) dissolve in water. They usually do not produce toxicity in the body since they flush out of the body with fluid elimination.

Important Functions of Vitamins

As connectors of organic functions, vitamins are known to improve metabolism, help prevent disease, and even retard the aging process. It probably will not surprise you to learn that the best sources of vitamins are found in vegetables, seeds (including nuts, whole grains, and legumes), and fruits.

God is so amazing and wise! He told Adam and Eve to eat bountifully the vegetables, seeds (nuts, whole grains, and legumes), and fruits created on the third day. The Creator knew plant life contains nourishment found in all six classes of nutrients. These same foods are important to our health and well being today.

CHOICES THAT DIMINISH THE BENEFITS OF VITAMINS

Cooking and Destruction of Enzymes

High temperatures weaken or destroy the nutrients in healthy foods. Enzymes are the life forces found in food. They prompt the nutrients to do their work in the body. The destruction of enzymes begins at 107° F and is completed by 122° F. The boiling point of water is 212° F. Therefore, boiling completely kills the life force in foods. Also, when foods are boiled, the most beneficial vitamins are lost in the water and disposed of in the kitchen drain.

Baking generally is done at 350° F, also weakening the nutritive value of plant life. Even a "slow oven" is at a temperature of 225° F or higher.

Foods are made from the four basic elements of nitrogen, carbon, oxygen, and hydrogen. Each food has a specific configuration of these elements. Our bodies contain the enzymes needed to digest foods in their proper configurations. However, foods also have a heat liable point where their configurations are changed. When the heating process drastically changes the foods' configurations, enzymes in the body are unable to adequately digest them, and the foods can actually become toxic.

Cooking and Weakening the "Body of Light" Within Foods

Each day billions of cells in our bodies are in the process of dying and being replaced by new cells all throughout the body. It has been estimated that within a year, each of us becomes a whole new person through this process.

A disturbing thought is that our bodies are, for the most part, dependent upon the nutrients we put into our systems to manufacture the new cells. When we ingest cooked, processed foods in our systems, the cells do not have good materials for the construction process. With our poor Standard American Diet, it is no wonder we have so many sick and dying people in our society! If we would eat foods closer to the way God created them, we would see a turnaround in our health as a nation.

Raw plant life contains live enzymes, which are matched perfectly to the enzymes in our cells. As we ingest raw vegetables or fruits, the live enzymes enter the body and are magnetically, and supernaturally, attracted to the very cells lacking their nutrients. Enzymes give the cells the construction materials needed to reproduce stronger cells rather than weaker, sicklier ones. Only God could ordain such a wonderful miracle to occur!

Also, when we eat pure, raw plant foods, their live enzymes cause the forward-spin and reverse-spin of the electrons to align and create a burst of pure light, referred to as a "body of light." This body of light helps repair damaged DNA in a cell.

God provides a beautiful foreshadowing of this truth from the Hebrew language. In biblical Hebrew, which originally had no vowels, the consonants in the word for "light" (אר) and "mouth" (פה) when combined are the same as the letters in the two words used for "heal" (*rapha* רפא or *raphah* רפה). Even the language of the Old Testament paints a picture that foods with a body of light, taken through the mouth, will heal. Therefore, the ingestion of live enzymes found in pure, raw plant life is a major factor in the difference between health and sickness. If we choose live plant foods created by God, in the natural states in which He created them, we actually ingest the light that can maintain, strengthen and heal our bodies.

Fresh vegetable juices are composed of live enzymes. (Fresh fruit juices are as well, yet they also contain an abundance of sugar and should be diluted.) If fresh juices are ingested on an empty stomach, the enzymes go to the cells immediately without going through the process of separating the fiber in digestion. To avoid an overload of sugar, it is better to sip, rather than gulp juices.

Also, raw seeds, including nuts, are an excellent source of fiber and protein, and they make wonderful snacks. We are told in scripture that one Sabbath *Jesus was going through the grainfields, and his disciples began to pick some heads of grain, rub them in their hands and eat the kernels* (Luke 6:1). We certainly could do well to follow this example given by Jesus' disciples.

Since most people prefer cooking foods, lightly steamed is an acceptable way of cooking vegetables to retain nutrients. However, keep in mind that enzymatic action will be weakened. To steam, place the vegetables in a stainless steel steamer with a small amount of water for a short time. Thinly sliced foods are ready within five minutes. When cooking legumes, it is best to bring them to a boil, then cook slowly at low temperatures.

Canning
High temperatures are used in the canning process, and nutrients are destroyed. In addition, canned foods often are filled with preservatives and additives. It is best to avoid buying canned foods whenever possible. Fresh foods are always best, and quick-frozen foods are second best. Dried foods are also acceptable in limited amounts, though not preferred.

CHOICES THAT DIMINISH THE BENEFITS OF ALL SIX CLASSES OF NUTRIENTS

In the name of progress, two processes have been developed in recent years that affect the overall nutritional content of foods. These two processes are forced ripening of foods and genetic modification (also called bioengineering or genetic engineering.)

Forced Ripening of Foods
In Ecclesiastes 3:1,2 we read that *there is a time for everything, and a season for every activity under heaven. . . a time to plant and a time to uproot.* A basic principle of life is that after seeds are planted their crops grow, ripen, and are harvested. For each aspect of food production, there is a specific time.

However, in the name of progress, food companies harvest foods before they mature, and "help" them ripen quickly by forcing growth in artificial environments. The foods are then irradiated to ensure longer shelf life. When plants are not allowed to ripen naturally, their compositions are altered. For example, ripened vegetables and fruits generally leave an alkaline ash in the body, but ones that have not ripened leave an acidic ash. Modern methods of food production can cause chaos on the cellular structures in the body.

A return to scriptural admonitions would help improve our health and well being. Man simply cannot improve the things ordained by God. *There is a time for everything* and we should not try to hurry the things of God.

Genetic Modification/Genetic Engineering

When God spoke the wonderful plant life of the third day into existence, scripture decrees specifically that they were created *according to their various kinds* (Genesis 1:11). The cells of living things, plant and animal, contain a genetic material called DNA, which tells the cells how to develop and live. DNA, the genetic "blueprint" of the cell, gives plants and animals their different characteristics. From the time God created plants (and animals), His intention was that they would propagate *according to their various kinds*.

Recently, however, scientists have altered DNA in the laboratory and created new types of plants (and animals). For example, in an attempt to produce frost-resistant vegetables, "antifreeze" genes from fish are injected into vegetables. The results are mutant variations of foods, no longer growing *according to their various kinds*.

One of the leading goals of genetic engineering is to produce foods that are resistant to certain pesticides. Then, when those pesticides are sprayed on a field, everything but the genetically modified plants will die.

Besides the fact that the safety of genetic modification is questionable, the fact that it contradicts scripture makes it undesirable. God created the world to be a beautiful place filled with life-giving foods. I doubt that He could look at what is happening today to His wonderful creations and still say that it is *good* (Genesis 1:12).

In Summary

In summary, for the sake of our health we would do well to choose naturally home grown plant life, processed as little as possible. In addition, we should incorporate some raw plant life into our daily diets. Remember our goal is to eat foods as closely as possible to the way God created them.

SPIRITUAL APPLICATION

God has shown through the creations of the third day that there can be unity in diversity. Each creation is different, yet working together they provide what is necessary for life to exist. Each category is created for a specific purpose. None of these creations could support life alone. However, by working together they have made life possible throughout the history of the world. One of our primary goals in life should be to work with others in such a way that our diversity produces strength rather than weakness. It is a noble goal, and one that will glorify God. In Philippians 2:2-5 we read,

> *. . . then make my joy complete by being like-minded, having the same love, being one in spirit and purpose. Do nothing out of selfish ambition or vain conceit, but in humility consider others better than yourselves. Each of you should look not only to your own interests, but also to the interest of others.*

The apostle Paul strongly admonishes in Romans 12:18, *"If it is possible, as far as it depends on you, live at peace with everyone."* Just as we enjoy seeing our children relate to each other in love, it delights the heart of God when we walk in unity and love: *He will rejoice over you with singing* (Zephaniah 3:17).

It is understandable why God twice pronounced an affirmation on the third day of creation. As we live in unity despite our diversity, we can be assured that our Creator will indeed affirm that "it is good."

Dear God of all blessings,

Thank You for creating each person on earth different and unique. Please forgive us when we see our differences as barriers rather than building blocks. Help us to try in our daily lives to work together in unity for the sake of Your kingdom. Lord, we want to please You and to accomplish the purposes for which You created us. We desire to cause You to rejoice with singing over us.

In Jesus' name I pray, Amen.

MEMORY VERSE FOR CHAPTER THREE:

I am the vine; you are the branches. If a man remains in me and I in him, he will bear much fruit; apart from me you can do nothing" (John 15:5).

ASSIGNMENT(S) FOR CHAPTER THREE:

1) **Increase** the amount of **alkaline-ash** foods you consume by choosing **5-7 servings of vegetables (primarily non-starchy or low-glycemic).**

2) Also, include **2-3 servings of fruits** in your diet daily.

Although not substantiated through Scripture, modern research shows that fruits eaten alone pass quickly through the stomach (in twenty to thirty minutes). However, when combined with other foods, their presence in the stomach causes digestive juices to begin to spoil animal protein foods and ferment carbohydrates. A good motto for consumption of fruits is "eat them alone or leave them alone."

Remember: Your goal is to choose a large percentage (many nutritionists say 75%) of your foods from the alkaline-ash group.

3) **Decrease** the amount of food you eat from the **acid-ash group**. Since most vegetables from the seed category—**some seeds, most nuts, whole grains, and legumes**—leave an acid ash but are high in fiber, carefully choose **3-5 servings** from this category daily. Choose high-fiber, low-acidic foods.

4) **Consume 1-2 Tablespoons** daily of **cold-pressed vegetable oils** which are good sources of essential fatty acids.

5) **Include raw plant foods daily**, preferably with each meal.

DEVOTIONAL FOR CHAPTER THREE

Day One

Scripture Reading: Mark 4:30-34

Verse of the Day. . . *I tell you the truth, if you have faith as small as a mustard seed, you can say to this mountain, "Move from here to* *there" and it will move. Nothing will be impossible for you* (Matthew 17:20).

During his first missionary journey to China, Hudson Taylor traveled on a sailing vessel. The wind became very still, and the boat began drifting toward the shore of an island where a savage tribe of cannibals lived. The captain came to Mr. Taylor and asked him to pray for God's help. Mr. Taylor replied that he would pray only if the captain agreed to set the sails to catch the breeze.

The captain did not want to appear foolish to his crew by unfurling the sails when there was no wind. Again Mr. Taylor declared that he would pray for the boat only if the captain prepared the sails. Reluctantly, the captain agreed. After some time, the captain came into Mr. Taylor's stateroom and politely asked him to stop praying. The crew could hardly manage the vessel in the high winds that had arisen.

Often we find ourselves in a dilemma similar to the captain's. Seemingly impossible circumstances come our way, and reasoning supercedes our faith. Jesus used the example of the mustard seed to teach a lesson in faith. Today's scripture from Mark explains that although the mustard seed is the tiniest vegetable seed of all, it grows to be the largest garden plant. It grows so large, birds can perch in its branches. Jesus compares this to the kingdom of God. Even a little faith goes a long way in helping us grow in holiness and obedience. It is simply a matter of trusting God.

An elderly lady in our church had a simple, yet profound, way of describing faith. Billie Bonnette, or "Miss Billie" as she was called lovingly, expressed it in the following acrostic:

> **F**orsaking
> **A**ll
> **I**
> **T**rust
> **H**im

Faith the size of a mustard seed is all it takes, but we must unfurl those sails.

Application:

1) In which areas of your life do you have the most difficulties trusting God?
2) Why do you think this is so? Do you feel that you are more capable than God?
3) What are some ways you can begin to develop "mustard seed" faith?

PRAY the prayer found in Mark 9:24, ". . . *help me overcome my unbelief!"*

DEVOTIONAL FOR CHAPTER THREE

Day Two

Scripture Reading: Numbers 11:4-9; Luke 9:57-62; Philippians 3:13,14

Verse of the Day: *We remember the fish we ate in Egypt at no cost—also the cucumbers, melons, leeks, onions and garlic* (Numbers 11:5).

God miraculously provided for the nation of Israel while they were in the wilderness. When they needed something, God supplied it. Water gushed out from rocks when they were thirsty. Fire appeared at night and a cloud during the day when they needed guidance. Bread fell from the sky when they were hungry. Now they were allowing themselves to be influenced by "the rabble," or discontented ones, in the group. Instead of gratitude for what they did have, they complained about what they did not have. Suddenly, they desired the foods they had eaten in Egypt.

The fact that they missed the foods they had enjoyed in Egypt was not wrong. The foods they mentioned provide a list of delicious, healthy foods. The problem was that they were so busy looking back, they could not receive the blessings of God's provisions at that time. Miracles were all around them, yet they complained. The Israelites were so focused on returning to the things of the past, they missed the gifts of the present.

In Luke 9:62, Jesus reminds us that when we begin to walk with the Lord, if we turn back, we are not fit for God's kingdom. Paul confirms this in Philippians 4:13,14 when he admonishes that to receive God's blessings we must leave the past behind. Leaving the past behind is often difficult, but it is necessary in order to live abundant lives daily.

Cucumbers, melons, leeks, onions, garlic—securities, happy memories, sad memories—what is it that keeps us from enjoying the gifts of the present because of bondage to the past?

Application:

1) What are some of the good things that keep you looking back to the past?
2) What are some of the bad things?
3) Does the past, in any way, keep you from living fully in the present?
4) If so, what can you do to put the past in its proper perspective?

PRAY and thank God for the past experiences that shaped who you are today. Thank Him that He is the great *I AM*, which means He is the God of the past, the present, and the future.

DEVOTIONAL FOR CHAPTER THREE

Day Three

Scripture Reading: Leviticus 23:9-14; Romans 8:22-25; I Corinthians 15:20

Verse(s) of the Day: *When. . . you reap a harvest, bring to the priest a sheaf of the first grain you harvest. He is to wave the sheaf before the Lord so it will be accepted on your behalf. . . On the day you wave the sheaf, you must sacrifice. . . to the Lord* (Leviticus 23:10-12).

Sacrifice is a word that often evokes a negative thought in our minds. However, sacrifice is essential for living as a Christian. Our scripture reading for today explains the origin of one of the annual festivals celebrated by the Jewish nation. When they harvested the grain crop they were to present a sheaf of it to God. A sheaf was a bundle of grain held together by a cord or band. Once the sheaf was presented to the Priest, he would wave it before God on their behalves.

This was considered a sacrifice because they were not to eat it, or even make bread from it, until they had presented this bundle from the first harvested crop. Barley was probably the grain presented on this day because it was the first to ripen.

In Romans, Paul says that believers have the firstfruits of the Spirit. In response to God's wonderful gift, we are to offer the sacrifice of our lives to Him. Romans 12:1 admonishes us to *offer our bodies as living sacrifices, holy and pleasing to God*. Amazingly, when we make lifestyle choices beneficial to our health we actually are offering a sacrifice to God.

However, the most wonderful example of firstfruits in the Bible is the resurrection of our Lord and Savior, Jesus Christ. He became the firstfruits of the dead. Those who accept His sacrifice on the cross of Calvary, and believe in His resurrection, will never have to die in the spiritual sense.

Several years ago an airplane crashed in frigid waters near Washington's National Airport. A friend saw the wreckage shortly after it happened. A rescue helicopter began pulling survivors onto the lift ladder. Suddenly, a man dove into the water, hoisted five people onto the ladder, then disappeared beneath the waves. None of the five people knew the man. He had given his life for people he did not know.

Jesus gave His life for us, yet He knew us with all our sins and faults. Let us offer a sacrifice to Him of the best harvest of our lives, not merely what is leftover.

Application:
1) What are you willing to offer to God as a sacrifice?
2) Will you ask Him to show you the way to live sacrificially?

PRAY and thank God for the fact that Jesus is our firstfruit offering.

DEVOTIONAL FOR CHAPTER THREE

Day Four

Scripture Reading: Matthew 13:24-30; Matthew 25:31-46

Verse of the Day: *Let both grow together until the harvest. At that time I will tell the harvesters, "First collect the weeds and tie them in bundles to be burned; then gather the wheat and bring it into my barn"* (Matthew 13:30).

We live in a world of deceit. On April 27, 1989, officials in Italy passed a mandatory seatbelt law for motorists. A psychiatrist devised a way to make money through deception. He invented a "security shirt." It was nothing more than a white T-shirt with a diagonal black stripe. The "security shirt" deceived policemen into thinking motorists were wearing seatbelts.

Today's scripture tells us how an unknown Palestinian farmer was deceived. This story parallels also the dilemmas Christians encounter in life. The farmer in the parable planted a field full of good wheat seed. While his workers were sleeping, the farmer's enemy came and sowed tares among the wheat. *Tares* are darnels, poisonous weeds that grow about the same height as wheat. Rabbis consider them to be distorted kinds of wheat.

When the plants grew and began to produce grain, the workers recognized the poisonous plants among the good wheat. The difference was recognized by what each plant produced. The farmer told the workers to leave them until the final harvest. At that time the poisonous plants would be destroyed. In Matthew 25:41-46, Jesus compares the fate of unbelievers and those unkind to the Jewish nation to that of the tares. Destruction will be the end result.

Even Believers have to live in an evil world. Like the wheat, Christians must co-exist among the tares. This parable clearly shows that the enemy is the cause of evil. He tries constantly to sow weeds in our lives to choke out the fruit we would bear for Christ. Notice that the enemy planted the weeds when the workers were asleep. Satan takes advantage of every moment we are not on guard.

It is important to realize that the workers knew the difference between wheat and tares through the seeds they produced. Can others look at our lives and immediately recognize to Whom we belong?

Application:
1) What is being produced in your life that identifies you as a Christian?
2) What tares do you recognize most in your life?
3) When and how do you think the enemy plants them there?

PRAY and ask God to reveal to you any tares that may be growing in your life.

DEVOTIONAL FOR CHAPTER THREE

Day Five

Scripture Reading: Deuteronomy 32:1-10

Verse of the Day: *Keep me as the apple of your eye. . .* (Psalm 17:8).

It was the Sunday before Thanksgiving. Our church's flower committee had prepared a beautiful holiday arrangement for the communion table. The cornucopia, surrounded by autumn leaves, was filled with colorful fruit. After the conclusion of the worship service our young daughters and I waited for my husband who was counseling some parishioners. As a pastor's family, we were accustomed to waiting but this session seemed to be unusually long.

I recognized that our daughters, who had been patient, became restless as it was long past time for lunch. Reluctantly, I reached into the beautiful display on the table to get a piece of fruit for each of them, vowing that I would replace it before the evening service. That satisfied them, but I kept looking at the fruit. The desire for the large red apple in the middle overcame me. As I reached for the apple and took a big bite, my husband walked into the sanctuary. I had been caught!

We got into the car and I continued munching on my "stolen" delight. I finished eating it right down to the core. My husband's car window appeared to be open, so I decided to toss it out his window. (By the way, I only "littered" with the apple core because I knew it would decompose quickly and return to nature.) Just as I hurled it, he turned to look at me, and I threw the core right into his eye. Thankfully, it only stunned him without injuring him.

Later I recounted the story to a friend who is known for her humor. Her immediate response was, "I know you want to be the 'apple of his eye' but that is not how to do it."

A study of the phrase, *apple of the eye*, reveals that many years ago people thought that the pupil of the eye was solid. They named it the "apple," believing that it was responsible for vision. Due to the importance of vision, the phrase came to refer to anything of value.

The scripture for today reveals that God refers to His children as the *apple of His eye*. Do you realize that God treasures you that much? Moses uttered these verses found in Deuteronomy 32 just before his death. He tried to convey to God's people how important they were to Him. He proclaimed they would be the *apple of His eye* forever.

Application:
1) Do you have any idea how much God loves you?
2) Do you realize that the God of the universe loves you as though you were the only person in the world?
3) Does the depth of your love for Him prove that He is the apple of your eye?

PRAY and thank God for the way He loves and treasures you.

DEVOTIONAL FOR CHAPTER THREE

Day Six

Scripture Reading: Galatians 5:16-26

Verse of the Day: *Thus, by their fruit you will recognize them*

(Matthew 7:20).

Today's scripture reading paints a graphic portrait of the two contrasts in life. Each person is controlled either by the Spirit of God or by the evil one. Paul, in this letter to the Galatian church, calls the attitudes and actions of the sinful person *acts of the sinful nature.*

In contrast, he calls the attitudes and actions of the redeemed person the *fruit of the Spirit.* Jesus explains in Matthew 7:20 that the manifestation of this fruit is the way to recognize whether or not a person is of God.

The *fruit of the Spirit is love, joy, peace, patience, kindness, goodness, faithfulness, gentleness, and self-control* (Galatians 5:22). This beautiful list of attributes is the full life that Jesus refers to in John 10:10 when He said, *"I have come that they might have life and have it to the full."*

The *fruit of the Spirit* can be divided by attributes into three groups, each with a different emphasis. The attributes in the first group—*love, joy, peace*—concern our relationship with God. Those in the second group—*patience, kindness, and gentleness*—relate to our relationships with other people. The attributes in the third group—*faithfulness, goodness, and self-control*—regulate the conduct of our personal Christian lives.

Paul refers to all of these attributes in the singular rather than the plural by calling them *fruit* instead of "fruits." Actually, they are different facets of the same category, comprising a unit. The *acts of the sinful nature* war against each other by striving to be the most dominant. The *fruit of the Spirit* work together bringing fullness and balance to the life of the believer. When our relationship with God is strong, we live our lives as God intended, and our relationships with others will be affected positively.

Perhaps we can take a lesson from the giant redwood trees in California that rise as high as three hundred feet above the ground. Unlike other trees, water and nutrients are not taken in through the root system to reach the leaves and branches, but rather, they are drawn by gravitational pull from above the trees. Likewise, may our nourishment for the *fruit of the Spirit* come from above!

Application:

1) Which of the three groups of fruit do you need most in your life presently?
2) Since the fruit are interdependent upon each other, are you aware of any problems within the other two groups that could be causing a lack in your area of need?

PRAY and ask God to reveal to you anything in your life that could be blocking the flow of His Spirit.

DEVOTIONAL FOR CHAPTER THREE

Day Seven

Scripture Reading: Matthew 9:18-38

Verse of the Day: *Then he said to his disciples, "The harvest is plentiful but the workers are few"* (Matthew 9:37).

This narrative occurred early in Jesus' ministry. He already knew the heartache of not having enough disciples to meet the needs of the multitudes that followed Him. God could have chosen to help the masses in many different ways. However, He chose to reach the world, both then and now, through His disciples.

What an awesome privilege! What a grave responsibility! God's compassion for the world must be lived through us.

My parents live in the rural area of my hometown several hours from my current home. I love to visit them. It seems that when I walk through their back door every muscle in my body relaxes. One of my favorite things to do while there is to help my father pick ripe vegetables in his garden. After all his hard work planting, fertilizing, watering, and weeding I am allowed the fun of helping him reap the harvest.

Last summer my father was in a serious car accident. Since internal injuries kept him from being able to harvest his garden, the neighbors on either side of my parents came daily to pick the vegetables for him. Without those wonderful neighbors, my father would have lost his garden.

Losing vegetables is one thing. Losing the souls of people is another. Jesus saw the multitudes and had compassion on them. He longed for people to help harvest the souls He had reached through His teaching and healing ministry.

When I go to visit my parents, my father has already done all the hard work. I simply enjoy harvesting the fruits (and vegetables) of his labor. Similarly, when it comes to sharing the gospel, my heavenly Father has done all of the hard work. He created each person, sent Jesus to die as the redeeming sacrifice, and convicts of sin through the Holy Spirit. Now He asks that we join in the fun of helping with the harvest!

One thing I have learned from my father's garden is that if the garden is not picked when ripe, the harvest is lost. Jesus pleads for us to work while souls are ripe so the harvest will not be lost.

<u>Application</u>:

1) Where do you see yourself in the garden of life? Are you a harvester or a spectator?
2) Is there anything in this world that is more important than helping Jesus harvest souls? What should be your response to your answer?

PRAY and ask the Father to send more workers into the fields.

(My father died shortly after the writing of this devotional)

CHAPTER FOUR

The Fourth Day of Creation

(Genesis 1:14-19)

14 And God said, "Let there be lights in the expanse of the sky to separate the day from the night, and let them serve as signs to mark seasons and days and years, 15 and let them be lights in the expanse of the sky to give light on the earth." And it was so. 16 God made two great lights—the greater light to govern the day and the lesser light to govern the night. He also made the stars. 17 God set them in the expanse of the sky to give light on the earth, 18 to govern the day and the night, and to separate light from darkness. And God saw that it was good. 19 And there was evening, and there was morning—the fourth day.

With the account of the fourth day scripture moves into the second triad of the creation order, commencing the second half of the creation week. The four fundamental elements of **light, air, water** and **earth** had been created, and now were ready for their intended use. Each fundamental element was carried to its ultimate completion during the second triad of creation.

The light created on day one was permanently settled in the creations of the fourth day. When God said, *"Let there be lights"* (Genesis 1:14), the Hebrew word used for *lights* was *meorot* (or *ma'owr*) which means "a luminous body or luminary." Literally in this passage God refers to a place where lights would reside, or light holders. A similar word is used for lamps and candlesticks throughout scripture.

On day one God summoned light, *owr*, into being. On the fourth day, He created *ma'owr*, the holders of the light. On this day, specific places were provided to serve as centers of radiation for the first fundamental element, light.

Genesis 1:14 pinpoints the location of these radiators of God's light, *in the expanse of the sky.* The Hebrew word for *sky, raqiya,* means "the expanse, or visible arch of the sky." In His wisdom, God created the world by first bathing the universe in His light and happiness then later creating heavenly bodies—the sun, moon, and stars—to serve as permanent receptors of that light.

Not only were the heavenly bodies receptors of divine light, they were created for distinct functions. These functions are listed in the concluding words of Genesis 1:14b,15: . . . *to separate the day from the night, and let them serve as signs to mark seasons and days and years, and let them be lights in the expanse of the sky to give light on the earth.*

I. <u>SEPARATE THE DAY FROM THE NIGHT</u>

Daytime and nighttime are vital to the welfare of plants, animals, and man. Daytime provides sunshine needed for growth and health. Plants need sunshine for photosynthesis to occur. Animals need sunshine for physical health. Man needs sunshine for both physical and mental well being. However, as necessary as sunshine is to all of life, continuous sunshine would be both monotonous and unhealthy.

Therefore, nighttime has its purpose also. The rest that accompanies nighttime is vital for the health and growth of plants, animals, and man. Plants take periods of relaxation from their vital processes in what is referred to as "vegetable sleep." Most plants fold their leaves and droop as nighttime approaches, indicating preparation for a time of rest.

Almost every animal species, with the exception of wild beasts, slumbers during the shadow of night's darkness. Man also is dependent upon rest and sleep to renew mental and physical energy.

In His infinite wisdom, God knew that both day and night were essential. Therefore, on the fourth day He made the provisions necessary for their sustained existence.

II. SIGNS

What is the purpose of a sign? When riding down the highway, if you see a sign on the side of the road, you know that its purpose is to convey information. The creations of the fourth day convey life's most crucial information—the story of redemption. The Hebrew word used here for *signs* is *'oth,* which means "markers or indicators."

In Psalm 19:1 David exclaims, *"The heavens declare the glory of God; and the skies proclaim the work of his hands."* Throughout history, God used the sun, moon, and stars for signs as indicators of His glory and redemption story. Numerous miracles and significant events have been and will continue to be associated with these heavenly bodies.

A brilliant star appeared during the time of Jesus' birth (Matthew 2:2). We are told in Matthew 24:29 that just prior to the return of Jesus to earth . . . *the sun will be darkened, and the moon will not give its light; the stars will fall from the sky and the heavenly bodies will be shaken.* In speaking about the same event, Luke 21:25 records, *"there will be signs in the sun, moon, and stars."*

The end of the world is characterized in II Peter 3:10 by the fact that . . . *the heavens will pass away with a roar; the elements will be destroyed with fire.* Then, in II Peter 3:13, we are assured that *we are looking for a new heaven and a new earth, the home of righteousness.*

The idea of the heavens declaring the glory of God goes back to the dawn of creation. In the stars we find the entire story of God's plan to redeem mankind. We are told in Isaiah 40:26, *"Lift up your eyes and look to the heavens; Who created all these? He who brings out the starry host one by one, and calls them each by name. Because of His great power and mighty strength, not one of them is missing."*

Also, Psalm 147:4 teaches that God *determines the number of stars and calls them each by name.* Since God deliberately ordained the number of stars and assigned each of them a name, the meaning of their names conveys God's purposes for creating them. What a beautiful thought that God not only created the world as a whole, but each component individually. As we look at the millions of stars in the sky, it is significant to realize that they were created one by one and named with an intended purpose in God's heart.

Since God named the stars when He created them, their names were already in place before He created Adam and Eve. Adam was given the privilege of naming the animals, but God had already named the stars. The names of the stars and the significance of the constellations were well known to the first of mankind.

In fact, the Jewish historian, Josephus, as well as ancient Persian and Arabian writings, attribute the oral tradition of the names of the stars to Seth, the son of Adam and Eve. This knowledge was passed down continually through the generations.

The actual recording of the names of the constellations is attributed to Enoch. Known as the Great Scribe, he was an early descendant of Adam who recorded sacred wisdom, particularly pertaining to astronomy: *Enoch, the seventh from Adam, prophesied about these men: "See, the Lord is coming with thousands upon thousands of his holy ones to judge everyone . . . "* (Jude 1:14,15).

The principle character of what is believed to be the oldest book of the Bible, Job, lived not long after Noah and the flood. The author was familiar with the constellations, and referred to them in his writings. The names of two groups of stars, Pleiades (a group of stars in the constellation now named Taurus) and Orion (a sidereal sidepiece of Taurus), are mentioned in Job 38:31.

Job refers to the annual pathway of the sun called the Mazzaroth (now called the Zodiac) in Job 38:32. Then in Psalm 19:4-6 the sun is compared to a bridegroom running a course through the heavens like a champion. John the Baptizer in John 3:25-32 refers to Jesus as the Bridegroom who came from heaven. Paul, in Ephesians 5, confirms this by comparing Jesus' relationship with the Church to that of a Bridegroom and His bride.

Many of the original Hebrew names given to the stars and passed down orally have been lost in antiquity. However, even the modern names and symbols of the twelve major constellations correspond to the story of redemption. Each constellation, along with the stars in its sidereal sidepieces, gives a dramatic, symbolic presentation of the gospel as shown by E. W. Bullinger in his book,

The Witness of the Stars. The comparison is correlated in three groupings of constellations through which the Sun (Son), who is the heavenly Bridegroom, runs His course in the heavens. These groupings are as follows:

A. The Advent of Jesus

The names of the first four constellations, or signs, correspond to the redeeming work of Jesus. These constellations begin with **Virgo**, "the Virgin," bringing forth the Messiah; then **Libra**, "the scales relating to the price of redemption," depicting the cost the Savior would have to pay to redeem mankind; and thirdly, Scorpio, "the attack of the enemy." In the group of stars comprising **Scorpio**, a "strong-man" [Jesus] is wrestling with a serpent [Satan] who is reaching for the crown of the "strong-man." The scorpion is stinging his heel, but he is treading on the scorpion [Genesis 3:15]. The fourth sign in this group of constellations is **Sagittarius**, which means "the gracious one." This entire constellation could be compared to Jesus, *the offspring of the woman*, who gains victory over Satan and his followers, the offspring of the serpent [Genesis 3:15].

B. The Redeemed

The names of the middle four constellations correlate to the redeeming work of the Savior in relation to the church, those who have accepted His gift of redemption. **Capricorn** is pictured as a goat with the tail of a fish. Throughout the Bible the goat represents a sacrificial animal, and the symbol of the early church was a fish. Beautiful imagery comprises this constellation! Jesus is the sacrifice (goat), and those who accept the sacrifice become part of the universal church (fish).

The second constellation in the middle quadriad is **Aquarius**, which means "the water-bearer." Throughout the New Testament, water refers to the Holy Spirit. Jesus told the woman at the well in John 4:14, ". . . *whoever drinks the water that I give him will never thirst. Indeed, the water I give him will become in him a spring of water welling up to eternal life.*" The ultimate example of this occurred on the day of Pentecost when God's spirit was poured out and the early church was born.

Pisces, the third constellation in the group relating to the church, literally means "the fish (multitudes) of those who will follow." Pisces is pictured as two fish with their tails tied together, corresponding to the vast body of believers who have received the water of life through the centuries.

The last constellation in this second quadriad is **Aries**, "the ram or lamb." Aries could be symbolic of Jesus, *the Lamb of God who takes away the sin of the world!* (John 1:29)

C. The Redeemer and the Final Judgment

The final four signs seem to depict the reigning Redeemer who will bring judgment upon the earth and put an end to the presence of sin. The first of these constellations is **Taurus**, "the bull." Taurus is pictured as a raging bull, representing judgment. The back end of the bull is coming out of the constellation Aires. As previously noted, Aries means "a lamb." Taurus is a magnificent sign, which could represent Jesus who came as *the Lamb of God* the first time, but will return in power and glory as the Judge of all the earth.

Gemini, the next constellation in the final group, means "the twins" and is depicted by two people. Some biblical scholars feel this constellation symbolically represents both the humanity and divinity of Jesus. Others believe that it is representative of the fact that Jesus, accompanied by His bride, the Church, will return to judge the earth.

The third constellation in this final group is **Cancer**, a crab. Although the meaning of Cancer is unclear, the major stars that comprise it help to give an explanation of its significance. Tegmine means "holding," Acubene means "sheltering or hiding place," and Ma'Alaph means "assembled thousands." The names of these stars, as well as the stars that comprise the sidereal sidepieces, lead to the conclusion that Cancer corresponds to heaven and the multitude of believers who will be sheltered there.

The final constellation in the third quadriad is **Leo**, "the lion who is hunting down its prey." Certainly this is a perfect ending to what many consider to be the gospel in the stars. In Revelation 5:5 Jesus is referred to as *the Lion of the tribe of Judah*.

I conclude this section with a description of the three sidereal sidepieces that accompany Leo. The first, Hydra, is pictured as a serpent and is so large it extends one-third of the distance around the circle of heaven. Revelation 12:4 refers to the fact that Satan, who had been an angel originally, rebelled against God and convinced one-third of the angels, also called "stars" in this passage, to become his allies. They were then cast out of heaven.

The second sidepiece, Crater, represents a cup, bowl, or vial being poured out on Hydra. This corresponds amazingly to the vials of God's wrath, found in Revelation 14-16, which one day will be poured out upon Satan and those who follow him.

The final sidereal sidepiece is Corvus, pictured as a bird eating the flesh of the serpent, Hydra. It is written in Revelation 19:17-21 that the fowl of the air will one day devour the flesh of those who follow Satan.

Praise God for caring so much about mankind that He shows through the names of the stars and their symbols how to live in a relationship with Him. Truly, *the heavens declare the glory of the Lord!*

III. SEASONS

The receptors of light created on the fourth day not only separated night from day and served as signs in the heavens, they also were created as signs for the seasons. The word *seasons* has a dual meaning.

The Hebrew word for *seasons, mowed,* means both "a fixed time" (indicating annual returning periods) and "a solemn assembly, a feast."

A. "A Fixed Time"

The first meaning of season, "a fixed time," represents summer, autumn, winter and spring, the four seasons of the year. *As long as the earth endures, seedtime and harvest, cold and heat, summer and winter, day and night will never cease* (Genesis 8:22).

God created the world with balance. In the present calendar, each season begins with an equinox (when the sun crosses the equator) or a solstice (when the sun is at its greatest distance from the equator). The two equinoxes are the vernal equinox (around March 21st) and the autumnal equinox (around September 22nd). On these days, day and night are of equal length. The two solstices in the Northern Hemisphere are the summer solstice (around June 21st or

22nd) the longest day of the year, and the winter solstice (around December 21st or 22nd) is the shortest day of the year. In the Southern Hemisphere, the solstices are reversed.

The balance of the seasons brings a variety of temperatures, affecting every aspect of life. Cultivation of land, germination of plants, and hibernation of animals are related to various seasons of the year. King Solomon penned that there *is a time for everything, and a season for every activity under heaven* (Ecclesiastes 3:1).

As we progress annually from season to season, we progress also through the seasons of life. In fact, the analogy of the four annual seasons is often used as a parallel to the stages of life. For example, youth is referred to as the springtime of life, and the elderly are said to be in the wintertime of life.

Activities and tasks that add an interesting variety to life accompany every season. In addition, each season brings with it a diversity of foods unique to that season. This variance of foods and activities helps to make our lifestyles more balanced and healthful.

B. "A Solemn Assembly"

The second meaning of *season*, "a solemn assembly," refers to the observances of the feasts and festivals of Israel. The Jewish feasts were ordained to teach us about God and His redemptive plan for mankind. They not only look back to events in Israel's history, they also teach about the role the Messiah would play in redeeming and restoring man back to God.

God instructed that seven major feasts and three rest periods should be observed. In addition, several "minor" feasts also were recognized. One notable feast, Hanukkah (Chanukah) or The Feast of Lights, was added in 165 B.C. when Judas Maccabaeus rededicated the Temple. This rededication occurred after the Syrian king, Antiochus IV (Epiphaneses), defiled the Temple by sacrificing a pig on the altar. The Maccabees overthrew him and then attempted to relight the eternal light in the Temple. Although they could find only enough oil for one day's supply, miraculously their prayers were answered and the light burned for eight days. Although Hanukkah was not one of the original feasts enumerated in Leviticus 23, it was prophesied in Daniel 8:9-14. There is also scriptural evidence that Jesus observed Hanukkah: *Then came the*

Feast of Dedication at Jerusalem. It was winter, and Jesus was in the temple area walking in Solomon's Colonnade (John 10:22,23).

The three rest times in Israel's religious calendar that pay tribute to God's work through creation follow:

The weekly Sabbath (Genesis 2:2; Exodus 20:8-11; Leviticus 23:1-3)

The seven-year Sabbath Feast (Exodus 23:10,11; Leviticus 25:2-7)

The fiftieth year Sabbath Feast also called **Jubilee** (Leviticus 25:8-16).

The seven feasts pay tribute to God's redemptive work through Israel and memorialize how God has saved and preserved Israel as a nation.

Also, the feasts correspond directly with the life, ministry, death, burial, resurrection, promise of the Second Coming, and establishment of the millenium kingdom of Jesus. In addition, the birth of the church and prophecies concerning future events coincide with the feasts and festivals of Israel.

The seven Feasts, and their corresponding New Testament counterparts, are as follows:

The Feasts of Israel
Feasts Observed During the First Month *(Normally April)*

Passover (14th day) Leviticus 23:4-8	**Jesus was crucified on Passover** I Corinthians 5:7
Unleavened Bread (15th day) Leviticus 23:6-8	**Jesus was buried** Matthew 26:17; Matthew 27:57-60
First Fruits (Sunday after Passover Sabbath) Leviticus 23:9-14	**Jesus arose on First Fruits** I Corinthians 15:20-23

Feast Observed Fifty Days After First Fruits *(May or Early June)*

Pentecost (Feast of Harvest) **(Feast of Weeks)** Leviticus 23:15-25	**The Full Coming of the Holy Spirit;** **Beginning of the Church** Acts 2:1-47

Feasts Observed During the Seventh Month *(September)*

Trumpets (1st Day) Leviticus 23:23-25	**Foreshadows the Rapture** **of the Church** I Thessalonians 4:13-18
Atonement (10th Day) Leviticus 23:26-32	**Foreshadows The** **Tribulation** Revelation 6-19
Tabernacles (15th Day) Leviticus 23:33-44	**Foreshadows The** **Millenium** Revelation 20:1-6

How amazing! Even before the holy days were initiated, God had made provision for them from the beginning of time. The sun, moon, and stars were designed to be indicators of "a solemn assembly" observed in honor of God.

IV. <u>DAYS AND YEARS</u>

As used in Genesis 1:14, the sun, moon, and stars also refer to the accumulation of days and years, and are indicative of time in general.

To the ancient Hebrews, nighttime and sunrise marked days. The times of sacrifice were based on daybreak (Leviticus 7:15). However, for the Jews, day began at sundown, as soon as three stars were visible in the sky.

Days were organized into weeks, but a week was not considered a portion of a month or year. The purpose of the week was to indicate the time for the Sabbath Day, or Shabbat.

Years among the ancient Hebrews were lunar. The first day of each month began with the new moon.

Later, probably after Israel had been exiled to Babylon, the Hebrews began to use a solar year, based on the rotations of the sun. However, the old lunar year calendar continues to be used for religious observances.

Most of the world goes by what is known as the Gregorian Calendar, based on the Julian Calendar initiated by Julius Caesar over 2,000 years ago. In 1583 A.D., Pope Gregory adapted the Gregorian calendar that counts the years as starting from the birth of Christ. Based on the solar year, it measures time by how long it takes the earth to circle the sun.

Jewish people calculate the current year by counting the number of years from creation as recorded in the Torah. For example, the year 2,000 A.D. on the Gregorian Calendar corresponds to the year 5760 B.C.E. ("Before the Christian Era") or C.E. (Common Era or Christian Era) which the Hebrews believe is the length of years since the creation of the universe.

In fact, Jewish people have several calendars that are very much a part of their lives. The first is the sacred, or religious (lunar) calendar, with the New Year usually beginning with the new moon in March or April. Another is the civil (solar) calendar, with the New Year occurring in September. A third is the Gregorian (solar) calendar, with the New Year beginning in January.

Many people own Jewish-Gregorian calendars, which give both the Jewish and Gregorian date for each day. This calendar also gives the dates of civil holidays and Christian holidays as well.

Certainly it is clear that the sun, moon, and stars created on the fourth day serve diverse purposes. These luminaries help maintain the balance of life instituted by the Creator. The sun, moon, and stars also proclaim His glory and the story of Redemption to the entire world. In addition, they mark seasons, religious observances, and time in general.

NUTRITIONAL APPLICATION

I. a. DAY (PHYSICAL LIGHT)

The importance of light in the spiritual sense was presented in the second chapter. The importance of light in the physical sense is also vital to the body's health. Humans are the embodiment of light. In fact, it is documented that all living things both take in and give off light. Fritz-Albert Popp, a West German chemist and physicist, discovered that the cells of all living things radiate light.

The basic components of life are light, air, water, and food. Since light helps sustain life, it is logical that insufficient light will negatively affect life. An improper "light diet" actually can cause illness. In a real sense, health is determined, among other things, by a person's ability to take in and utilize light.

Even the energy within our bodies can be produced only with the aid of light. A car's engine must have fuel, oxygen, and a spark to create the internal combustion that makes the car run. In the same way, our bodies must have fuel (food), oxygen (air), and a spark (light) to ignite the process of metabolism.

Light Therapy

Light is used currently as "medicine." Studies are prolific concerning the positive effects of light on healing. Photodynamics, the term that is used to describe light therapy, is considered the wave of the future. Laser surgeries are replacing more intrusive types of surgeries. Light is used at Baylor University to kill viruses in the blood. Research offers hope that light therapy will combat cancer and other life-threatening diseases.

Natural Sunlight

Sunlight is our major source of light, warmth, and energy. It sustains not only life on earth, but also the earth itself. Sunlight provides plants with energy needed for photosynthesis. Plants in turn sustain the lives of animals and humans.

Energy from sunlight is transmitted to earth in the form of electromagnetic waves. The visible portion of this electromagnetic spectrum, containing all the colors of the rainbow, is one of the most important keys to human function.

The light of each new day seems to bring a new beginning. With the brightness of each day comes a heightened sense of energy.

Nothing can replace the benefits of natural sunlight. Various studies have proven conclusively that artificial light does not provide the same benefits as natural sunlight. One research study measured the life span of laboratory animals kept under different light sources. Mice living under pink or white fluorescent lighting lived on the average 7.5-8.2 months, while those living under natural light lived 16.1 months.

This study led to the development of full spectrum fluorescent lighting. Although full spectrum lighting is superior to other forms of fluorescent lighting, it is not as healthy as natural sunlight. As we discovered how to produce artificial light, we became disconnected from natural sunlight.

Benefits of Natural Sunlight

The benefits of natural sunlight for the health of humans are varied and numerous. Some of the benefits are as follows:

- Sunlight stimulates the immune system.
- Sunlight activates the synthesis of Vitamin D and therefore the absorption of calcium and other minerals.
- Sunlight kills bacteria, viruses, and other infectious agents.
- Sunlight lowers blood pressure.
- Sunlight increases the efficiency of the heart.
- Sunlight reduces cholesterol.
- Sunlight assists in weight loss. (Sunlight stimulates the thyroid gland, increasing metabolism and burning calories. Farm animals living outdoors do not fatten as easily as those living indoors.)
- Sunlight increases the level of sex hormones.
  (A study at Boston State Hospital found that male hormone levels increased 120% when men were exposed to natural sunlight. Another laboratory study proved that estrogen is most efficient when a woman is exposed to the ultraviolet wavelengths of the sun.)

- Sunlight regulates not only our physiology but also our emotions.
- Sunlight taken in through the eyes affects the brain and every cell of the body. (As light enters through our eyes, it goes through the retina to the pineal gland. Neurotransmitters are produced which influence the function of the endocrine system. Mood, sleep, and even the timing of the biological clock are all affected.)
- Sunlight determines the value of the foods we eat. Foods manufactured directly from sunlight are more healthful. The lower we eat on the food chain (plants) the more vibrant our foods will be. The higher we eat on the food chain (animal products) the less quality we will receive from the energy of light.

Since the benefits of sunlight are numerous, we should make an effort to be exposed to sunlight at least a portion of each day. God created us to benefit from sunlight. However, He also expects us to use wisdom in how and when we are exposed.

CHOICES THAT DIMINISH THE BENEFITS OF SUNLIGHT

From the dawn of creation man was meant to enjoy the benefits of the outdoors. Adam and Eve were given a beautiful garden as their home. In today's society, that has changed somehow. We seem to feel that staying indoors is normal. We are in buildings all day long—homes, schools, offices, factories, and stores. As a result we have become overweight, pale, and lacking of energy.

Symptoms of light deprivation have become epidemic. Some of these include the following:

- Irritability
- Fatigue
- Illness
- Lowered immune functioning
- Hypersomnia
- Depression

- Alcoholism
- Suicide

Scientists at the National Institute of Mental Health have pinpointed an emotional disorder, Seasonal Affective Disorder (SAD), characterized by drastic mood swings and depression. They found that this disorder usually arrives in winter and lasts until spring.

Behaviors of those affected include increased eating (especially carbohydrates), increased sleeping, decreased interest in sex, weight gain, personality change, and withdrawal from people.

It was concluded that this disorder is the direct result of light deficiency, particularly sunlight. This disorder is also called "sunlight starvation," and it is estimated that 25 million people in the United States suffer from SAD. Special lighting is available to help with this disorder and can be found at many home improvement stores.

Another way the benefits of sunlight are destroyed is by misuse, or overexposure. Enjoying fresh air and sunshine is one thing, but baking our bodies by lying in one position for a long period of time is another. The rays of direct sunlight can cause damage to the skin. Therefore, we must cautiously choose to be outside when the rays are not as hot and direct. Since the rays of the sun are most intense between 10:00 a.m. and 2:00 p.m., early morning or late afternoon hours are best.

Begin with short periods of time and build up until you feel you are enjoying a healthy amount of sunlight. As with other parts of The Creation Diet, balance is the key.

I. b. NIGHT (SLEEP)

William Shakespeare beautifully expressed, "Sleep knits up the raveled sleeve of care." Certainly stress-filled days are mended by the gift of peaceful rest and sleep.

Sleep was designed to be a time for restoration of the body's natural balance, homeostasis. Depending on age, the body requires that approximately one third of the twenty four-hour day be spent in sleep.

Sleep is somewhat of a mystery. For many years it was believed that sleep was a period of quiet inactivity. Now it has been proven that many vital processes occur in the body as we sleep, such as the following:

- Brain waves slow.
- Blood pressure lowers.
- Muscles relax.
- Activities of the heart and lungs somewhat decrease.
- Blood circulates throughout the body to deliver oxygen and nutrients.
- Toxins are carried away by the blood and lymph systems.
- Hormone production from the pituitary gland increases.
- Enzymes activate protein production to repair damaged cells and tissues.
- Immune cells are activated to fight free radicals.
- Many growth processes occur during sleep.
- Dreams occur, allowing the mind to deal with unresolved anxieties and fears.

The benefits of sleep are essential to the overall well being of a person. So the natural question that arises is, "How much sleep is enough?" The answer varies from person to person depending on many circumstances. However, generally speaking, the following is suggested:

> Babies require 10 hours of sleep.
> Children require 8 hours of sleep.
> Adults require 7 hours of sleep.

Except in the case of babies, approximately 1/3 of the day is required for sleep.

Sound sleep is absolutely vital to healthy living. God intended it to be that way. From various scriptures we are assured that God wants His creations to enjoy restful sleep. In Psalm 4:8 the Psalmist said, " *I will lie down and sleep in peace, for you alone, O Lord, make me dwell in safety.*" Also, Psalm 127:2 promises that. . . *he grants sleep to those he loves.*

CHOICES THAT DIMINISH THE BENEFITS OF RESTFUL SLEEP

God intends for His creations to enjoy the benefits of restful sleep. However, on the average, Americans are getting 20% less nighttime sleep than a century ago. It is estimated one in every four Americans is sleep deprived and over 40 million suffer from some form of chronic sleep disorder.

According to statistics, over 24,000 persons die in accidents every year by falling asleep at the wheel. One in every three fatal truck accidents is the direct result of sleepiness.

As shocking as these numbers are, it is even more shocking to realize that many sleep disorders are due to poor lifestyle choices. When the body is out of balance, sleep is one of the areas that is affected drastically.

The following are only a few of the things that often leave a wake of insomnia and restlessness rather than restfulness:

- Caffeinated or alcoholic beverages
- Medications (many pain relievers contain caffeine)
- Oxygen deficiency from shallow breathing
- Tension and anxiety
- Lack of exercise
- Vitamin and Mineral Deficiencies (especially B-complex, calcium/ magnesium)
- Food allergies
- Overeating
- Toxin forming foods
- Too much noise
- Too much light
- Uncomfortable environmental temperatures
- Restrictive clothing
- Uncomfortable mattress
- Conditions such as viral infections, chronic fatigue, PMS, and menopause

In looking at the list, we easily can note that most of the deterrents to restful, natural sleep are choices we make. It is amazing how taking a few steps to promote good sleep can make a tremendous difference in our health, our mental attitude, and our total well being!

Developing nighttime rituals before going to bed can mean the difference between a night of restful sleep and a night of tossing and turning. A good night's sleep begins long before we ever actually lie to rest.

Besides avoiding the deterrents to sleep as listed above, suggestions for improving overall sleep are as follows:

- Begin to relax before going to bed through the use of nighttime rituals in order to convey to your body that you are preparing for sleep. For example, you may choose to wash your face, put on comfortable sleepwear, take a warm bath, perform light stretching exercises, and pray.
- Listen to your body. Do not attempt to stay awake when your body is telling you that it is ready for sleep.
- Go to bed early. God made darkness for sleep. The dark hours before midnight are said to be the most beneficial hours of sleep. Even the rhythms of the body (mentioned in the beginning chapter) confirm this. During the hours of 8:00 p.m. and 4:00 a.m. the body is in the assimilation process, which means the body is absorbing the nutrients from digested food.
- Use the bed only for sleeping or enjoying intimacy with your spouse. Do not watch television (especially the nightly news), listen to loud or fast music, or do heavy reading that would make your mind more alert. Try to avoid concentration as this also keeps the mind too active to sleep.
- Keep a pad and pen or tape recorder beside the bed so you may record conveniently any thoughts you may have while in bed. This simple step will prevent you from being filled with the anxiety that you may forget something important by morning.
- Various aromas (such as lavender) promote sleep. Spray them on your pillowcase or burn candles that contain these relaxing scents before retiring.
- Avoid medications to promote sleep, as these can imbalance the body. If you feel you must take something, various natural

herbs are available as sleep aids. (The chamomile tea Grandma used to make for you is actually a wonderful choice.)

- Set your alarm, but try to cultivate the habit of waking up naturally instead of with an alarm. Awaking to an abrupt sound can produce an agitated state of mind.

- Arise at the same time regardless of how little sleep you have received. This practice helps the body get into a habit of waking and retiring at the same time daily.

- If you need more sleep than you are getting presently, begin going to bed fifteen minutes earlier. After your body has adjusted to that bedtime, go to bed fifteen minutes earlier. Keep doing this until you have found the right bedtime for you. Researchers have found that fifteen-minute blocks seem to be more effective at adjusting your schedule than larger periods of time.

- Try to take ten-minute rest periods (not necessarily sleep periods) throughout the day. These help to reduce stress and prepare the body for sleep.

- Don't worry! Give to God any concerns you have. Remember: . . . *he who watches over you will not slumber; indeed, he who watches over Israel will neither slumber nor sleep* (Psalm 121:3b,4). Your Creator will be up all night tending to your problems.

- Go to sleep at night looking forward to tomorrow, which has the potential to be the best day of your life: *How precious it is, Lord, to realize that you are thinking about me constantly! I can't even count how many times a day your thoughts turn toward me. And when I waken in the morning, you are still thinking of me!* (Psalm 139:17,18 TLB)

II. SIGNS

God revealed Himself miraculously through the signs of the *Mazzaroth*. The story of the redemption of mankind is told in the twelve constellations. God (the Father) loves each person He created so much that He came to earth as the "Strong Man" (Jesus) and died as the ultimate sacrifice for sin. He did this so that His special creations could have victory over the serpent, Satan.

God also loves each person He created so much that He (the Holy Spirit) indwells all who accept the gift of His sacrificial death. The Church was established as the means to equip and encourage those who have had this life-changing experience and to serve as a catalyst for helping others with spiritual needs. Believers who have accepted the victory of the "Strong Man" will live eternally in heaven.

In addition, God loves each person He created so much that He one day will bring final judgment upon the evil one and his followers. A wonderful time of peace will be established on earth for one thousand years. After that, this earth as we know it will be destroyed and the new heavens and earth will begin.

The signs of the *Mazzaroth* point to the fact that God (the Father, Son, and Holy Spirit) is in control of the beginning and end of life, and everything in between the two. Individually and cosmically, God is in control.

What does this have to do with nutrition? If you will recall, the beginning of The Creation Diet is about developing a relationship with God, the Source of light. The signs of the *Mazzaroth* point us to the Source of light. When we live in a relationship with God, we will have wisdom in the choices that produce health and vitality.

Those who have received and accepted the story of redemption as told even by the stars are transformed. The Holy Spirit resides in them. Their bodies actually become the dwelling place of God: *Do you not know that your body is a temple of the Holy Spirit, who is in you, whom you have received from God? You are not your own; you were bought at a price. Therefore honor God with your body* (I Corinthians 6:19,20).

This realization should make us want to develop the nutritional habits that promote health and honor God. The presence of the Holy Spirit empowers the believer to realize and implement the lifestyle choices that provide health and well being.

It is not an easy task, but it is possible. The daily requirement is that we die to the old habits and come alive to the beneficial ones. This becomes an act of worship to God, as a way to honor Him with our bodies: *Therefore, I urge you, brothers, in view of God's mercy, to offer your bodies as living sacrifices, holy and pleasing to God— this is your spiritual act of worship* (Romans 12:1).

How do we do this? Through a day by day, step by step, minute by minute process. It involves bringing to God every thought that is contrary to what is beneficial for us. It is living in a constant state of dependence upon Him: *Do not conform any longer to the pattern of this world, but be transformed by the renewing of your mind. Then you will be able to test and approve what God's will is—his good, pleasing and perfect will* (Romans 12:2).

He created us and has told the redemption story through the stars: *If there is a natural body, there is also a spiritual body* (I Corinthians 15:44). With the help of the "Strong Man" as displayed in the stars, we can make spiritual choices concerning our bodies. For after all: . . . *the body without the spirit is dead* (James 2:26).

CHOICES THAT DIMINISH THE BENEFITS OF SIGNS

The purpose of all creation, including the sun, moon, and stars, is to bring honor and glory to the Creator. As previously acknowledged, the various constellations and stars of the *Mazzaroth* tell the story of the Creator's unselfish love for His created ones. It is all about God and how we as humans can be given victory over the bondage of the evil one.

Satan has a counterfeit for every wonderful thing that God has provided. Therefore, it stands to reason that there would also be a substitute version of God's plan for the world as revealed in the stars. In fact, this perversion of God's story is so widespread, it is accepted as the norm among many people.

The signs of the *Mazzaroth*, or Zodiac, were intended solely to bring glory to God and to bring people into a relationship with Him. However, the story in the stars has become so perverted through the years, it is now used to glorify man-made, mythological deities and to attempt to tell fortunes. Astrology and worship of the sun, moon, and stars has taken the place of worshipping God and trusting His guidance. The Bible speaks clearly about the error of such practices, as evident in the following verses:

> *And when you look up to the sky and see the sun, the moon and the stars—all the heavenly array—do not be enticed into bowing down to them and worshiping things the Lord your God has apportioned to all*

the nations under heaven (Deuteronomy 4:19).

> *Let no one be found among you who sacrifices his son or daughter in the fire, who practices divination or sorcery, interprets omens, engages in witchcraft, or casts spells, or who is a medium or spiritist or who consults the dead. Anyone who does these things is detestable to the Lord...* (Deuteronomy 18:10-12a).

God never intended these purposes for the sun, moon, and stars. Scripture relates repeatedly that we are to trust God with our futures, not the stars. Satan is behind the practices of the occult. Any information he offers is likely to be distorted and dangerous.

Only God has a perfect plan for our lives. Only God knows the path we should follow to achieve His plan. Only God can redirect us when we get on the wrong path. Only God loves us that much!

- *The Lord is my rock, my fortress and my deliverer; my God is my rock, in whom I take refuge. He is my shield and the horn of my salvation, my stronghold* (Psalm 18:2).
- *When I am afraid, I will trust in you* (Psalm 56:3).
- *You saw me before I was born and scheduled each day of my life before I began to breathe. Every day was recorded in your Book* (Psalm 139:16 TLB).
- *Trust in the Lord with all your heart and lean not on your own understanding; in all your ways acknowledge him, and he will make your paths straight* (Proverbs 3:5,6).
- *You will keep in perfect peace him whose mind is steadfast, because he trusts in you* (Isaiah 26:3).
- *Therefore I tell you, do not worry about your life, what you will eat or drink; or about your body, what you will wear. Is not life more important than food, and the body more important than clothes? Look at the birds of the air; they do not sow or reap or store away in barns, and yet your heavenly Father feeds them. Are you not much more valuable than they? Who of you by worrying can add a single hour to his life?* (Matthew 6:25-27).
- *Therefore do not worry about tomorrow . . .* (Matthew 6:34).

III. a. <u>SEASONS</u>
A Fixed Time

The four seasons bring with them a variety of environmental changes, activities associated with these changes, and a broad diversity of vegetables, seeds, and fruits. The luscious melons of summer, apples and pumpkins of autumn, squashes of winter, and tender green vegetables of spring produce an interesting medley of foods to enjoy.

God provides a myriad of plant foods from which to choose, varying in type, taste, and color. Some categories of vegetables, seeds, and fruits are as follows:

Vegetables
Root vegetables such as potatoes, beets, carrots, turnips and sweet potatoes
Bulb vegetables such as onions, leeks and garlic
Flowering vegetables such as broccoli and cauliflower
Head vegetables such as cabbage and lettuce
Leafy vegetables such as parsley, kale, spinach, collards and various greens
Hanging vegetables such as tomatoes and peppers

Seeds
Seeds such as flax, pumpkin, sunflower and squash
Nuts such as almonds, pecans, walnuts, brazil nuts, peanuts, hazelnuts, pine nuts and pistachios
Whole Grains such as wheat, rice, barley, rye, millet, corn, oats, spelt and quinoa
Legumes such as kidney, pinto, soy, lima, navy and black beans; black-eyed and split peas and lentils

Fruits
Grown on vines such as grapes and kiwi
Grown on bushes such as blackberries, blueberries, raspberries, gooseberries, huckleberries and currants

Grown on the ground such as strawberries
Grown on trees such as pears, apples, oranges, lemons, grapefruits, peaches, plums, apricots, bananas, mangoes, avocados and olives.

Edible plants that adorn our plates are available in a rainbow of colors such as red, yellow, orange, brown, green, purple, pink and white. One rule of thumb is that the greater the variety of colors that comprise a meal, the more healthful the meal is. Another guideline is that the deeper or brighter the color of the vegetable, the more healthful it is. Rich-colored vegetables contain more phytochemicals, and thus more antioxidant qualities.

Unless they naturally grow white (such as potatoes), do not eat white foods. This rule includes sugar, bleached flour, white rice, man-made salt, shortening and all products made from them. The lack of color in these foods is the result of manufactured processing.

The closer we eat to the way God created plants, the healthier we will become. A portion of the plant life we eat daily should be raw. If God made it, eat it bountifully. If man processed it, eat it sparingly, or not at all.

God wants His creations to be blessed with an abundance of healthful foods. Genesis 2:16 records that . . . *the Lord God commanded the man, "You are free to eat from any tree in the garden; but you must not eat from the tree of the knowledge of good and evil."*

Many people hesitate to eat freely because of the fear of gaining weight. However, if we eat the foods God created, in the order He created them, and we eat them as closely as possible to the way He created them, we may eat abundantly and without fear.

Our Creator has blessed mankind with a wonderful assortment of vegetables, seeds, and fruits that accompany each season. A diet plentiful in **vegetables** (at least **5-7 servings** per day), **seeds (3-5 servings** per day), and **fruits** (**2-3 servings** per day) will promote health and deter a number of degenerative diseases.

Enjoy the four seasons. Also, enjoy the bountiful foods God has made available during each season. Long before it became a well-known cliché, God understood that variety is the spice of life. In His miraculous way, He made provision for variety.

CHOICES THAT DIMINISH THE BENEFITS OF SEASONS

"A Fixed Time"

Nutritionally speaking, the sun, moon and stars mark a season, or "a fixed time" that produces a variety of healthful vegetables, seeds, and fruits. These foods are available and they not only add diversity to our diets, they also help balance the types of foods consumed.

In the past, people depended on a variety of vegetables, seeds, and fruits to stay healthy. As recently as 50 years ago, people ate over twenty different types of vegetables. They grew what they ate and stored a supply for winter.

Today, people eat only about eight different vegetables including corn, peas, potatoes, green beans, head lettuce, green peppers, cucumbers, and tomatoes. We have become a generation of "picky" eaters.

The foods that most Americans prefer are fats, processed carbohydrates, caffeine, and sugar (including alcohol). Therefore, the same foods are eaten repeatedly. Since these foods do not nourish the body, they act as foreign substances in the body, which must be handled by the immune system. The body can become allergic to these foods, and in the process of trying to adapt to them, the body becomes addicted to them. If the cycle of allergy-addiction continues over a period of time, a host of degenerative diseases, as well as acute diseases, occurs.

The answer to this problem is simple. Eat a variety of foods available during the four seasons. Eat them in the order God created them. Eat them as closely as possible to the way He created them. Enjoy!

III. b. SEASONS
"A Solemn Assembly"

As previously noted the sun, moon, and stars were intended to mark the special feasts and holy days of the Lord, given to Israel. One may wonder how this relates to our physical well being. The answer can be found in what takes place bodily while we are in our mother's womb. The milestones during the gestation and birth of a human baby directly correspond to the seven feasts of Israel found in Leviticus 23 and the eighth feast, Hanukkah, added in 165 B.C.

As mentioned earlier, we are reminded that God . . . *saw me before I was born and scheduled each day of my life before I began to breathe* (Psalm 139:16 TLB). When we realize how directly our prenatal development coincides with the feasts of Israel, that verse takes on a new and wonderful meaning.

A summary of the feasts found in Leviticus 23 follows:

Feasts Observed During the First Month
Passover—14th Day (a one-day observance)—reminds us of the blood of the lamb placed on the door posts when the firstborn children of the Israelites were spared as the Death Angel passed through Egypt. The Jews place an egg on the Passover table to represent the new life granted by the sacrifice of the lamb in Egypt. **Unleavened Bread—15th Day (a seven-day observance)**—reminds the Jews that when God delivered Israel from Egypt they were instructed not to take time to let the bread rise in their hasty exodus. This feast commemorates leaving behind the old life and entering a new way of living.
First Fruits—the time varies, but it is always the Sunday after Unleavened Bread (a one-day observance)—celebrates the first crops of barley that were planted and harvested. First Fruits reminds the Jews how God has provided for them.

Feast Observed Fifty Days After First Fruits
Pentecost, Feast of Weeks, Feast of Harvest—50 days after First Fruits (a one-day observance)—distinguishes the end of the barley harvest and the beginning of the wheat harvest. Pentecost reminds the Jews to be thankful for the bountiful harvest. It also commemorates the giving of the law at Mount Sinai that took place on Pentecost.

Feasts Observed During the Seventh Month
Trumpets, also called Rosh Hashanah—1st Day (a one-day observance)—marks the beginning of the civil new year. This feast encourages the Jews to express joy and thanksgiving to God.
Day of Atonement, also called Yom Kippur—10th Day (a one-

day observance)—symbolizes the removal of sin from the people and the nation by an acceptable blood sacrifice. Day of Atonement is designed to restore fellowship with God.

Tabernacle—15ᵗʰ Day (a seven-day observance)—commemorates God's protection and guidance in the desert. The Feast of Tabernacles provides a means to renew Israel's commitment to God and trust in His guidance and protection.

Feasts Observed During the Ninth Month

Hanukkah, also called the Feast of Lights, and the Feast of Dedication—25ᵗʰ Day (an eight-day observance)—celebrates the rededication of the Temple in 165 B.C. and commemorates that the eternal light miraculously burned for eight days when there was only oil for one day. Hanukkah reminds the Jews of God's miraculous eternal light.

A Child is Born

Often the pre-natal terms used to describe a human being from fertilization to birth are zygote, morula, embryo, and fetus. However, the biblical word used for an unborn baby (*babe*) is the Greek word *brephos*, which means "unborn infant, infant, (young) child."

The average pregnancy lasts 280 days and is counted from the first day of the menstrual cycle before conception. Amazingly, as Zola Levitt has written, the major landmarks of a baby's development follow the cycle of the eight feasts. In other words, the days between the landmarks of a baby's development are the same number of days as those between the feasts of Israel!

The "ideal" Jewish year would begin with the new moon on the first day of the first month and would occur on the spring equinox, March 21ˢᵗ. Taking an average length pregnancy of 280 days beginning on March 21ˢᵗ, the following scenario would develop:

Ovulation—On the 14ᵗʰ day of the first month, ovulation would take place. Ideally, this would happen on **The Feast of Passover,** which is celebrated on the 14ᵗʰ day of the first month. As previously stated, an egg is used on the Passover table as a symbol of new life. How appropriate, since the appearance of the female egg (ovulation) has the potential of also producing a new life!

Fertilization—On the 15th day of the first month, fertilization would occur. This corresponds with **The Feast of Unleavened Bread**, which takes place the day after Passover. The fertilization of the egg must occur within 24 hours or the egg will pass on through the body. Likewise, The Feast of Unleavened Bread occurs within 24 hours of Passover.

Implantation—The time that the fertilized egg travels down the fallopian to the uterus varies anywhere from two to six days. The time is indeterminate, but always within a week. During this time, the fertilized egg must be implanted in the wall of the uterus for a pregnancy to occur. This time frame corresponds with **The Feast of First Fruits**. First Fruits represents the barley seed, which has been planted and produces a full harvest. Since it is observed on the Sunday after Unleavened Bread, First Fruits is also an indeterminate time, but always within a week. It varies from year to year, depending on which day of the week Unleavened Bread occurs. However, since it must be within the same week, it could occur anywhere from two to six days.

Embryo/Fetus—Fifty days after the baby is conceived, all the organs of the body are in place. Every system that is found in a fully-grown human has been formed, and the embryo has progressed from a single cell to millions of cells. Fifty days is the milestone when most medical personnel change the terminology of the baby from embryo to fetus. The baby is small, but very definitely a human being.

Likewise, **The Feast of Pentecost** when the church was established took place fifty days after First Fruits. Although small, it was very definitely the body of Christ.

Perfected Hearing—Although all the systems and senses of the baby have formed already, they remain in the process of being further developed and perfected. The baby has been hearing sounds for quite some time. However, medical research confirms that by the 1st day of the seventh month, the baby is able to make a distinction between the sounds he or she hears. **The Feast of Trumpets** occurs on the 1st day of the seventh month. What a glorious sound for the baby to be able to distinguish first as the shofar trumpet heralds this feast!

Acceptable Blood—While in the womb, the baby receives

oxygen and other nutrients from the mother, delivered through the umbilical cord connecting the baby to the placenta of the mother. Waste products are also disposed of through this same system. However, the fetal blood, which carries the mother's oxygen through the baby's system, must change before birth. The hemoglobin requires transformation in order to have the ability to carry the oxygen the baby will receive when it is born and is breathing on its own. The blood must become "acceptable" to receive oxygen upon birth, even though it will continue to carry the mother's oxygen until then. This change occurs on the 10th day of the seventh month. Miraculously, this change in the blood corresponds with **The Feast of the Day of Atonement**. People in the nation of Israel presented animals to be used by the High Priest as blood sacrifices to ensure forgiveness of their sin. If the blood of the animal sacrifices were deemed to be "acceptable," they would provide new life free from the bondage of the past life of sin. Likewise, when the blood of the baby is acceptable to receive oxygen, it can live at birth free from the placenta of the mother.

Developed Lungs—By the 15th day of the seventh month the lungs are developed enough to function. This day directly corresponds with **The Feast of Tabernacles.** In the baby, the cells that line the alveoli (air sacs) of the lungs begin to secrete a soapy substance called "surfactant," which keeps the air sacs from collapsing. Depending on how well developed the lungs are, the baby could breathe outside the womb should a premature delivery occur. In the Bible, the Tabernacle is considered the house of the spirit of God. In biblical Hebrew, the word *ruwach* is the same for *spirit, breath,* and *air.* How appropriate that the lungs which carry the breath of air would be developed fully by the spiritual day, The Feast of Tabernacles!

Birth of the Baby—Again taking the Jewish sacred calendar placed on the "ideal" year, the 280 days of gestation would culminate on December 25th, the accurate date of **Hanukkah, The Feast of Dedication,** or **The Feast of Lights**. The Source of light creates each life that is born into this world. What a beautiful realization that even before we were born we symbolically accomplished each of the feasts of the Lord!

CHOICES THAT DIMINISH THE BENEFITS OF LIFE ASSOCIATED WITH SEASONS
(A Solemn Assembly)

Abortion

The most obvious choice that would destroy the benefits of the life developed according to the seasons or "solemn assembly" of the feasts of Israel is to end a life before it is born. A look at the original meaning of the word "life" puts the seriousness of this choice in clear perspective.

The Hebrew word for the noun "life" is *chay* and it means "alive." It directly derives from the Hebrew verb *chayah* whose definition not only means "to live," but also "to make alive, to keep alive, give (promise) life, let live, surely save life, be whole."

This was God's original intention for life. "Live and let live" is much more than a saying. It is God's will as revealed in scripture.

Medical communities define abortion as "the end of a pregnancy before viability" (being sufficiently developed to maintain life outside the uterus). Since the legalization of abortion by the United States Supreme Court in 1973, over 40 million abortions are known to have taken place. Each day over 4,000 lives are ended in America alone through various forms of abortion.

Human Cloning

For years the idea of human cloning was considered a science fiction fantasy. Now it has become a reality, sparking heated debates concerning its ethical and political ramifications.

The three types of cloning are embryo cloning (also called embryo splitting), reproductive cloning (also known as nuclear transfer, somatic cell nuclear transfer, or adult DNA cloning) and therapeutic cloning.

Embryo cloning removes one or more cells from a fertilized embryo. The removed parts are then implanted and have the potential of becoming a child. This process yields multiple embryos with identical DNA.

Reproductive cloning produces a duplicate of the existing animal or person. DNA is removed from an ovum (egg). Then, DNA taken from the cell of an adult is inserted by either injection or electrofusion into the ovum. This infused ovum (referred to as a "pre-embryo") is implanted in a womb and allowed to develop into a child identical to the adult who donated the DNA.

Therapeutic cloning initially begins with the same procedure as reproductive cloning. However, stem cells are removed from the "pre-embryo" to produce either tissue or a whole organ for transplant back into the DNA donor. The pre-embryo dies in the process.

It is evident that any type of cloning bypasses God's beautiful design by which the major milestones of human development correspond to the feasts of Israel. In addition, it interferes with God's plan to create uniquely and individually each person in his or her mother's womb! (Psalm 139:13)

Poor Lifestyle Choices during Pregnancy

The complexity of developing from two cells into the trillions of cells that comprise a human body is a process that requires a broad spectrum of nutrients. Each baby is absolutely dependent upon his or her mother for oxygen, vitamins, minerals, and all other nutrients.

Every choice the mother makes before and during pregnancy is crucial. The mother's lifestyle choices will affect the developing baby, the mother herself, and the actual birth. Decisions made before pregnancy are also important since some essential nutrients and/or toxins can be stored in the tissue of the mother.

The following are but a few of the choices that diminish the benefits of the full life God intended for each of His creations. Just as they affect those who already have been born, they are especially crucial in the development of those who are yet to be born.

Malnutrition

Failure to eat in the way God intended can lead to deficiencies in the six main nutrients and the numerous micronutrients. Deficiencies in these nutrients can result in loss of life through miscarriage, as well as a host of birth defects and disorders. The Creation Diet promotes health at every age and every stage of development.

Caffeine

On the average, American women drink 28 gallons of caffeinated beverages a year, coffee being the most concentrated.

One study found that a cup of coffee, 5 cups of tea, or 4 cans of cola per day doubled the risk of miscarriage.

Research has confirmed that caffeine produces birth defects in laboratory animals. Studies have not proven whether caffeine produces birth defects in babies, but research does conclude that caffeine interferes with the normal growth of babies including low birth weight and head circumference. This possibly could be due to the fact that caffeine decreases the blood flow through the placenta.

Although a safe dose has not been established, women who consume 300 mg. or more (3-5 cups of coffee) per day present the highest risk. In the later stages of pregnancy caffeine disrupts sleep and other vital activities of the baby.

Tobacco

Tobacco smoke contains thousands of chemicals, many of which are toxic. One such chemical, carbon monoxide, constricts vessels to the placenta, interfering with the oxygenation of the blood and, in a real sense, suffocating the baby.

Smoking also depletes the tissues of many essential nutrients. Therefore, it not only suffocates the baby, it subsequently can lead to starvation. Smoking not only results in smaller birth weight and smaller babies in general, it also presents a greater risk of death soon after birth.

Alcohol

Alcohol crosses the placenta freely and directly exposes the developing baby to toxicity. Unfortunately, alcohol travels in the baby's bloodstream in the same concentration as that of the mother. However, the immature development of the baby's nervous system, liver, and kidneys do not allow adequate detoxification of the alcohol. As a result, it stays in the baby's body much longer, wreaking havoc as it travels.

Fetal Alcohol Syndrome, a result of maternal alcohol consumption, directly affects the growth and development of the baby. Babies with this condition are shorter, weigh less, and have small heads. They often have facial malformations, joint and limb abnormalities, and heart defects as well.

Babies afflicted with Fetal Alcohol Syndrome frequently have mental retardation, poor coordination, and emotional problems. Unfortunately, the mother's choice to consume alcohol during pregnancy will negatively affect these babies for the rest of their lives. No safe amounts of alcohol consumption during pregnancy have been determined.

Drugs (Illicit, Prescription, Over the Counter)

Like alcohol, other drugs cross over the placenta directly into the bloodstream of the baby. Since drugs often deplete nutrients in the user, the baby is robbed of the life-giving nutrients that would ensure proper growth and development.

The possibility of Sudden Infant Death Syndrome is increased with the use of drugs. In addition, there is additional risk of birth defects while using drugs.

As with caffeine, tobacco, and alcohol, no safe limits of drugs have been established. Therefore, all drugs, unless closely supervised by medical personnel, should be avoided, especially during pregnancy.

IV. <u>DAYS AND YEARS</u>

The days and years of life, determined by the sun, moon, and stars, accumulate over a period of time. Scripture teaches that our Creator placed each of us on earth for a specific period of time. Therefore, we as individuals have a predetermined accumulation of days and years that comprise our lives.

In Job, what many consider the oldest book of the Bible, we read some of the most poignant words regarding this subject: *Is there not an appointed time to man upon earth? Are not his days also like the days of an hireling?* (Job 7:1 KJV)

We read further in the book of Job that *man's days are determined; you have decreed the number of his months and have set limits he cannot exceed* (Job 14:5).

David was quite clear that God has predetermined a number of days for our earthly existence. In Psalm 39:4,5 he pleads, *"Show me, O Lord, my life's end and the number of my days; let me know how fleeting is my life. You have made my days a mere handbreadth; the span of my years is as nothing before you. Each man's life is but a breath."*

David also asks that God would *teach us to number our days aright, that we gain a heart of wisdom* (Psalm 90:12).

Solomon refers to a set number of days on earth in Ecclesiastes 8:15 when he speaks of *the days of the life God has given him under the sun.*

This same affirmation is continued in the New Testament. Luke records in Acts 17:26,27 that *from one man he made every nation of men, that they should inhabit the whole earth; and he determined the times set for them and the exact places where they should live. God did this so that men would seek him and perhaps reach out for him and find him, though he is not far from each one of us.*

The writer of Hebrews states that *it is appointed unto man once to die and after this the judgment* (Hebrew 9:27 KJV). The Greek word for *appointed* in this verse is *apokeimai*, which literally means "to be reserved; to be laid up."

Many scientists believe that the average life span of human beings should be around one hundred and twenty years. Dr. Leonard Hayflick, a scientist at the University of California in San Francisco, discovered in the early 1950's that human cells are able to reproduce themselves only a certain number of times. He estimated that number to be around fifty cell divisions, which would place the human life span around one hundred and twenty years.

In the first book of the Bible we read God's words stating, *"My Spirit will not contend with man forever, for he is mortal; his days will be a hundred and twenty years"* (Genesis 6:3). In this verse God pronounced the length of time He would allow people in Noah's day to live before He sent the flood. However, it seems that in this verse the Creator also hid a truth now being "discovered" by modern scientists and longevity researchers.

The Process of Aging

For many years it was believed that the accumulation of *days and years* solely accounts for aging. To some degree it does, but not entirely. Things do age naturally with the passing of time. Webster defines aging as "the process of becoming old, or older." Aging is a universal process associated with all living things.

However, the rate of deterioration that accompanies aging is not universal. It is an individual rate, depending on a variety of personal factors and circumstances.

A more recent definition of aging from the research community is "a monumental progressive deficiency disease." Yes, aging is a degenerative disease as well as an accumulation of *days and years*.

Although we cannot control the normal process of aging (the accumulation of *days and years*), we can control the accelerated process of aging (progressive deficiency disease). The majority of degenerative diseases are acquired rather than genetic. Therefore, the majority of maladies that accompany aging are unnecessary, and even in most cases reversible.

Free Radical Damage

The war raging inside our bodies on the molecular level is the primary cause of the diseases that accelerate the aging process. Although other causes may be discovered in the future, free radical damage is one aspect of deterioration that has been identified already. Over sixty different conditions and diseases, many that previously were considered age-related, have been associated with free radical damage in the body.

The following are some of these conditions and diseases: wrinkles (caused by collagen deterioration), joint stiffness, arthritis, rheumatism, varicose veins, heart disease, stroke, hardening of the arteries, Alzheimer's, Parkinson's, cataracts, hemorrhoids, kidney and liver disorders, and cancer. In 1954, Dr. Denham Harman, M.D., Ph.D., the first pioneer Emeritus Professor of Medicine at the University of Nebraska College of Medicine, exposed the connection between free radical damage and aging. Dr. Harman states, "Very few individuals, if any, reach their potential maximum life span; they die instead prematurely of a wide variety of diseases — the vast majority being free radical diseases."

As was explained in the beginning chapter of The Creation Diet, free radicals are molecules that are missing an electron from the pair of electrons that travel around the nucleus of the cell. In their unstable condition, these unbalanced molecules collide with healthy cells trying to steal one of their electrons. After the healthy cells have lost an electron, they also become scavenger free radicals. A chain reaction begins. The fats inside the damaged cells turn rancid, proteins become rusted, membranes are pierced, and the genetic code of the DNA is perverted. Eventually the damaged cells die.

Free radicals are produced in the body by natural and unnatural means. The natural production of free radicals is the by-product of the combustion of oxygen in the mitochondria of the cells when we breathe.

The unnatural production of free radicals is the result of poor nutrition, stress, pollution, cigarette smoke, alcohol, caffeine, various other drugs (illicit, over-the-counter, and prescription), and radiation (including televisions, microwave ovens, computers, etc.) Alkaline-acid imbalances in the body and free radical damage are produced mutually by these factors. All diseases can be attributed to an overload of toxins that overwhelms the lymph system, the center of the immune system.

Antioxidants to the Rescue

A healthy immune system is able to withstand the onslaught of free radicals, allowing them to be neutralized by antioxidants. Antioxidants are chemical compounds that stop the formation of free radicals, stabilize them, and destroy them if necessary. Antioxidants then help to repair the damage caused by free radicals.

It is easy to see that we need an abundant supply of antioxidant nutrients. Antioxidants include Vitamins C, E, beta-carotene (becomes Vitamin A in the body), and the B-complex vitamins. Bioflavonoids, although not true vitamins in the strictest sense, are sometimes called Vitamin P because they aid in the absorption of Vitamin C.

Although bioflavonoids are not produced by the body, they can be obtained from the foods we ingest or through supplemental forms. Pycnogenols, found in green and black teas, the bark of certain pine trees, and grape seeds and skins are antioxidants that help to eliminate free radicals and aid in the absorption of other antioxidants. Minerals such as copper, selenium, zinc and magnesium also fight free radical damage. Certain amino acids are considered antioxidant nutrients due to the fact that they stimulate the natural antioxidants of the body. In the future, many more antioxidants probably will be identified.

Since antioxidants are so important for health and vitality, you may be wondering how we can get them. **The primary way to intake antioxidants is by eating foods that are rich in antioxidant properties**. The vegetables, seeds (including nuts, whole grains, and legumes), and fruits found in plant life contain high concentrations of antioxidants.

However, with the aging process certain factors begin to affect how nutrients are processed in our bodies. Malabsorption problems keep nutrients from being absorbed properly from the gastrointestinal tract. As we age, the amount of stomach acid needed for digestion decreases, the assimilation of nutrients lessens, and the systems of the body slow and become less efficient.

These factors, coupled with the loss of nutrients through the processing of foods, necessitate the addition of supplements to fortify our bodies' defenses against free radical damage. Herbs, vitamins, minerals, essential fatty acids and supplements that stimulate enzymes are a necessary part of health and nutrition.

Some Suggestions for Supplements to Slow the Aging Process

People are unique individuals. Therefore, daily habits are unique depending on the choices made by each individual. It is difficult to devise a "prescription" that is right for everyone. Various disorders require different nutrients for correction.

Generally speaking, the following list includes some essential nutrients that are available in supplemental form. As with any decision regarding health, it would be wise to consult with a health professional about these choices.

Whole food multivitamins-minerals that contain the RDA requirements for vitamins, minerals, and trace elements
The following should be added if they are not included in the multivitamin tablet:
B-Complex (which includes 50 milligrams of B6, 500 to 1,000 micrograms of B12, and 1,000 micrograms of folic acid)
Vitamin E (not to exceed 1,000 IU)
Vitamin C (500 to 1500 milligrams)
Beta Carotene (10 to 15 milligrams)
Coenzyme Q-10 (30 milligrams)
Chromium (200 micrograms)

Calcium (500 to 1500 milligrams)
Magnesium (200 to 300 milligrams)
Selenium (50 to 200 micrograms)

A few other anti-aging supplements that might help those who are middle aged or older:
Digestive enzymes (one with each meal)
Ginkgo (40 milligrams)
Garlic (as directed)
Essential Fatty Acids (such as fish oil and/or flax seed oil.) **Do Not** consume fish oil if you are on a medication to thin the blood.

Some people require hormonal supplementation, which must be determined after testing by medical professionals. The above list names a few of the basic supplements and whole foods that help fight free radical damage. With wise lifestyle choices, the degenerative diseases that come with the accumulation of *days and years* can be deterred.

CHOICES THAT DIMINISH THE BENEFITS OF DAYS AND YEARS

Age can be a blessing rather than a curse. Many years ago the magazine <u>Good Business</u> recorded an interesting thought: "Years should be regarded as an asset. Come to think about it, God must be very old. But has anyone ever suggested that the years must have robbed Him of His ability to hold the stars in their courses, and that it is about time He was retiring and making a way for someone younger?"

Age does have many advantages. The wisdom that has been acquired through the years can lead to choices that ensure a fulfilled and satisfied life.

A person's age is determined more by his or her outlook on life and physical vitality than the actual chronological number of years. Perhaps all of us know young people who are old and old people who are young.

When the Bible speaks of the death of King David it says that *he died at a good old age, having enjoyed long life, wealth and honor* (I Chronicles 29:28).

David had not led a perfect life by any means. However, the lessons he learned in life can teach us how to make choices that lead us to *a good old age, having enjoyed long life, wealth and honor.* Failure to learn these lessons will rob us of the fulfillment and satisfaction God designed to accompany the accumulation of *days and years.* Some of the choices that rob us of the benefits of *days and years* are the following:

• **Poor Food Choices**

As previously mentioned, poor food choices lead to a depravation of essential nutrients and antioxidants. These nutrients are needed to fight the free radical damage that causes disease and accelerates aging.

David knew that his strength and vitality were dependent upon food that would nourish his body. He also knew that good food would help to keep him young: [God] *satisfies your desires with good things so that your youth is renewed like the eagle's* (Psalm 103:5).

• **Worry (Stress)**

David learned that God would help him overcome even the worst circumstances in life: *When I am afraid, I will trust in you* (Psalm 56:3). . . . *in God I trust; I will not be afraid. What can man do to me?* (Psalm 56:11)

Worrying causes stress to the body and mind, and stress causes imbalances in every hormonal system of the body. These imbalances can lead to disease and premature aging.

Stress is a fact of life that cannot be avoided. We live with everyday pressures that are the natural result of our stress-filled world. In addition, stressful events occur over which we have no control. Some of these are death of a loved one, divorce, loss of a job, accidents, and sudden illnesses.

Although stress cannot be avoided, worrying can be. We can choose to trust God as David did, and not allow stress to fill us with anxiety.

David was a king who had many enemies as well as many admirers. Often his enemies tried to kill him and rob him of power. He also had made poor decisions that led to heartache and trials. However, in the midst of it all he chose to trust God rather than to worry.

- **Physical Inactivity**

Lack of physical activity suppresses the immune system and leads to a host of illnesses and conditions. The main age-related markers in the human body are bones, muscles, metabolism, and the cardiovascular system, and all these components are affected positively by exercise. Physical activity protects and improves them.

David was the king. He could have chosen to live a life of ease. Instead, we find that David was acquainted with physical activity. He recorded, *"man goes out to his work, to his labor until the evening"* (Psalm 104:23). It was David who realized that God rewards every man according to his work (Psalm 62:12).

Swift and Company once had an advertisement that read, "A man buried in work is usually very much alive." Although we do not need to be buried in our work in order to stay very much alive, we do need to stay physically active.

- **Mental Inactivity**

Lifetime learners have an exciting edge in life. Learning new things actually helps to slow the aging process of the brain. A quote from the Wall Street Journal several decades ago stated, "No one is ever too old to learn, but many people keep putting it off." Our Creator gave us a wonderful gift by not determining a certain age where learning must cease.

David realized the importance of lifetime learning. He pleaded with God to help him remain teachable. Whether he realized it or not, David had found one of the greatest assets to his longevity: *Show me your ways, O Lord, teach me your paths; guide me in your truth and teach me* . . . (Psalm 25:4,5). *Teach me your way, O Lord; lead me in a straight path*. . . (Psalm 27:11). *Teach me your way, O Lord, and I will walk in your truth*. . . (Psalm 86:11). *Teach me to do your will*. . . (Psalm 143:10).

- **Lack of Purpose in Life**

Many people begin to give up on life as they age. Failure to have a purpose for living is one of the primary reasons for the loss of health, vitality, and eventually life. Many people "die" long before their deaths. Lack of purpose leads to existing rather than living.

People who refused to lose their purposes for living as they aged have given some of the greatest contributions in every area of life. Nearly two-thirds of the greatest deeds ever accomplished were by people over the age of sixty. These include victories in battles, writing of great literature, creations of art and music, inventions, and new discoveries. Goethe completed writing <u>Faust</u> at eighty. Likewise, Verdi wrote an opera at eighty. Oliver Wendell Holmes was writing magnificent essays at ninety. Many of the authors who wrote about the Holocaust concluded that the people who survived the death camps were those who had a reason to live.

King David continued to have a purpose for living, even when he was aged: *Even when I am old and gray, do not forsake me, O God, till I declare your power to the next generation, your might to all who are to come* (Psalm 71:18). David never lost sight of his purpose for living, which was to teach others about God.

* **Loss of Hope**

Sophocles once said, "It is hope which maintains most of mankind." How true, for it is hope that keeps us living, not simply "being." Those who have lost hope have lost life. Those who have lost life consciously or unconsciously choose to age and then die.

At the very beginning of <u>The Creation Diet</u>, it was revealed that God began creation with light and happiness. A relationship with the Source of light, which leads to happiness, is at the very core of <u>The Creation Diet</u>. This includes the element of hope.

In Proverbs 13:12 Solomon wisely observes, *"Hope deferred makes the heart sick."* Ezekiel's vision of a valley filled with dry bones gives us insight into the reason people had died: *Then he said to me: "Son of man, these bones are the whole house of Israel. They say, 'Our bones are dried and our hope is gone'. . ."* (Ezekiel 37:11).

David had learned in his lifetime that hope strengthens, preserves, and keeps a person alive in the fullest sense of the word: *Be strong and take heart, all you who hope in the Lord* (Psalm 31:24). *May your unfailing love rest upon us, O Lord, even as we put our hope in you* (Psalm 33:22).

- **Isolation**

The feeling of connection, or belonging, is important at every age. However, as people grow older it often becomes physically more difficult to participate in activities outside the home. They can begin to lose their sense of connection, or belonging, with other people in the world around them. A feeling of isolation sets in and with it a despair that can hasten the aging process.

A recent study showed that heart attack victims are 50% more likely to have a second heart attack within six months if they are experiencing the feeling of isolation. If they live alone, they are two to three times more likely to die than their married peers. It has also been estimated that those who feel isolated are hospitalized for mental disorders five to ten times more frequently than those who have a sense of belonging.

David knew the importance of staying in fellowship with other people. He often referred to being in the company of others who also loved God: *I will praise you, O Lord, among the nations; I will sing of you among the peoples* (Psalm 108:3). *For the sake of my brothers and friends, I will say, "Peace be within you"* (Psalm 122:8). *How good and pleasant it is when brothers live together in unity!* (Psalm 133:1)

Sun, moon and stars. . . day and night, signs, seasons, days and years. . . what a powerful and wonderful message is conveyed by the creations of the fourth day!

SPIRITUAL APPLICATION

God is **omnipotent** (all powerful).
. . . For Thine is the kingdom, and the power, and the glory forever. Amen (Matthew 6:13 KJV).
. . . I heard what sounded like the roar of a great multitude in heaven shouting:
"Hallelujah! Salvation and glory and power belong to our God". . . (Revelation 19:1).

God is **omniscient** (all-knowing).
For He looketh to the ends of the earth, and seeth under the

whole heaven (Job 28:10,11 KJV).

O Lord, you have examined my heart and know everything about me. You know when I sit or stand. Even far away you know my every thought. You chart the path ahead of me, and tell me where to stop and rest. Every moment you know where I am. You know what I am going to say before I even say it (Psalm 139:1-4 TLB).

And even the very hairs of your head are all numbered (Matthew 10:30).

God is **omnipresent** (everywhere all the time).

You both precede me and follow me, and place your hand of blessing on my head.

. . If I go up to heaven, you are there; if I go down to the place of the dead, you are there. If I ride the morning winds to the farthest oceans, even there your hand will guide me, your strength will support me (Psalm 139:5, 8-10 TLB).

Perhaps the most concrete proof of these biblical truths can be seen in the sun, moon, and stars. The celestial bodies created on the fourth day demonstrate to mankind how big God is, and how small we are. Only God could have the power to create them, the knowledge to chart and sustain their courses, and the ability to display His presence through them.

It is difficult for our finite minds to understand the infinite mind of God. Job expressed it well when he said, *"The Almighty is beyond our reach and exalted in power; in his justice and great righteousness. . . "* (Job 37:23).

Isaiah recorded God as saying, *"As the heavens are higher than the earth, so are my ways higher than your ways, and my thoughts than your thoughts"* (Isaiah 55:9).

The supernatural wisdom of Almighty God, who has the **omniscience** to conceive of the sun, moon, and stars; the **omnipotence** to create them; and the **omnipresence** to keep them in their courses, is truly higher than our minds can fathom.

Can we even begin to imagine the power that hurled our planet through space at a velocity of 65,000 miles per hour? Can we conceive of the strength that created the sun 109.2 times bigger than the earth? Can we fathom the brilliance of the light that makes the moon glow with clear visibility 238,000 miles away from earth? Can we picture the creativity that fashioned millions of galaxies with over 200 billion stars in each one?

Yet as powerful, knowledgeable, and ever present as God is, He is a Creator who tenderly and compassionately loves each of His creations. He loves us so purely, it is hard for us as humans to comprehend.

Sun, moon, stars. . . omnipotence, omniscience, omnipresence. . . *The heavens declare the glory of God* (Psalm 19:1).

Dear God,

We worship and adore You. Truly You are the King of kings and Lord of lords.

We praise You for Your omnipotence. We praise You for Your omniscience. We praise You for Your omnipresence. We praise You because You are You. And, oh, how we love You!

In Jesus' name I pray, Amen.

MEMORY VERSE FOR CHAPTER FOUR:

The heavens declare the glory of God; the skies proclaim the work of his hands (Psalm 19:1).

ASSIGNMENT(S) FOR CHAPTER FOUR:

1) Spend time each day in the **fresh air and sunshine**. Gradually build up to **30 minutes per day** outdoors when the sun's rays are not direct.

2) Determine the amount of **sleep** your body requires, approximately **1/3 of the day (8 hours)**. If you presently are not getting enough sleep, begin the process of adjusting your bedtime by going to bed fifteen minutes earlier progressively until you are getting adequate rest.

3) Develop your relationship with God and participate in meaningful **religious observances**.

4) Choose servings of **vegetables (5-7), seeds (3-5),** and **fruits (2-3)** from a variety of colors. Take advantage of the seasonal foods that are available.

5) Determine to make **lifestyle choices** that will ensure **health and fulfillment** as you age. Remember that God created you with a purpose in mind, even before you were in your mother's womb. **Seek God's guidance daily**, finding your intended purpose as you progress through the seasons of life.

DEVOTIONAL FOR CHAPTER FOUR

Day One

Scripture Reading: Ephesians 4:23-32

Verse of the Day: *In your anger do not sin: Do not let the sun go down while you are still angry. . .* (Ephesians 4:26).

In his letter to the church at Ephesus, Paul lists the characteristics that follow a life-changing experience with the Lord. As we allow our minds to be transformed through His Spirit, we as believers find that we do the following:

v.25 Will not lie, but will tell the truth
v.26 Will deal with anger in an appropriate and timely manner
v.27 Will not give Satan any place in our lives
v.28 Will not steal, but will work hard so we can assist others
v.29 Will speak only what benefits others
v.30 Will not grieve the Holy Spirit
v.31 Will not have an attitude of ill will toward anyone
v.32 Will love, understand, and forgive others

God knows that there are times in life when circumstances anger us. Thus, He teaches in Ephesians 4:26, *"In your anger do not sin."* So the question arises, "When does anger become sin?"
The answer is found in the latter part of the same verse. Anger

becomes sin when we choose to hold onto it and refuse to deal with it. Anger that is not dealt with turns into resentment, and ultimately into unforgiveness. The Bible is specific that we *Do not let the sun go down while you are still angry* (v.26). We may experience some long nights as we deal with situations that have angered us, but it is vitally necessary to our spiritual well being that we do not "sleep on our anger."

Solomon admonishes in Proverbs 16:32, *"Better a patient man than a warrior, a man who controls his temper than one who takes a city."* With 700 wives and 300 concubines, he must have been speaking from experience.

Remember, "anger" is only one letter short of "danger." Do not let the sun go down with "danger" in your heart.

Application:

1) Is there unresolved anger toward another person in your heart?
2) Who is being hurt by that anger, you or the other person?
3) What do you think God would have you do about it?

PRAY and ask God to renew your mind through His Spirit so you can release anger to Him. He longs to free you from the binding influence anger has on your life!

DEVOTIONAL FOR CHAPTER FOUR

Day Two

Scripture Reading: Joshua 10:12-14

Verse of the Day: *So the sun stood still, and the moon stopped, till the nation avenged itself on its enemies, as is written in the Book of Jasher* (Joshua 10:13).

Few objects in the world have inspired awe and mystery as does the moon. As a child I gazed at the moon, imagining there was a man inside who watched everything I did. As a teenager I stared at the moon on a romantic summer's evening. As an adult I heard the immortal words of a tearful newscaster, "Ladies and gentlemen, man has landed on the moon."

Even as I write these words today, a total lunar eclipse is scheduled to occur tonight close to midnight. There is an excitement in the air as Americans plan to arrange their bedtimes around this event.

Of all the mystique and wonder that surrounds the moon, perhaps none is more remarkable than the account in today's scripture. The Book of Jasher was a collection of historical events put to music. In his songs, Jasher noted that Joshua prayed and asked that the sun and moon stand still. The nation of Israel needed extra light to avenge the enemies of God. Joshua's prayer was miraculously answered and the Amorites were defeated while it was still day.

With today's scientific knowledge of the universe, we are aware that the sun does not move, but rather the earth revolves around the sun. However, we should not allow the biblical terminology to diminish the importance of the miracle. Similar terminology is used even today when we talk about the sun rising and setting.

In whatever way God accomplished the miracle, the significance is that God answered Joshua's prayer and somehow provided a longer period of daylight for the army of Israel. Jasher's song declares, *"There has never been a day like it before or since, a day when the Lord listened to a man. Surely the Lord was fighting for Israel!"* (v.14)

God is always in control and He is always on the side of right. Whatever means are necessary to accomplish His purposes, He has the power to make them come to pass!

Application:

1) Thank God that whatever you are facing in life, He has the power to do whatever is necessary to accomplish His purpose through you.

Pray that just as the moon reflects the light of the sun, you can live in such a way that your life reflects the light of the Son.

DEVOTIONAL FOR CHAPTER FOUR

Day Three

Scripture Reading: Psalm 147:1-20

Verse of the Day: *He determines the number of the stars and calls them each by name* (Psalm 147:4).

We cannot begin to imagine the super-intelligence of God. Not only did He determine how many stars there would be in the universe, He created them and then assigned a name to each of them.

The concept of a "name" was very important in Bible times. A name did more than identify a person or an object, it also expressed the essence, the character, or the reputation of the person or thing. Therefore, when the Psalmist exclaims that God calls each star by name, we can be sure that each was given its name for a special purpose.

If God took the tender care to assign a significant name to each star, imagine how special His loving thoughts are toward His most treasured creations. . . each of us! David says in Psalm 139:17,18, *"How precious it is, Lord, to realize that You are thinking about me constantly! I can't even count how many times a day Your thoughts turn towards me. And when I waken in the morning, You are still thinking about me!"* (TLB)

I remember the time and care taken when we named our two daughters. Our first-born, "Meri Beth," was three days old before we finally confirmed her name. We had several different names under consideration, and we took into account the meaning of each of them. After much deliberation, we named her in honor of her two grandmothers, and changed the spelling so that her name literally means, "happy house of God." She certainly is that!

We knew we wanted to name our second daughter "Molly." However, the deliberation came in choosing a middle name to accompany it. Again, after researching the meanings of many different names, we chose "Melinda" which means "mild, gentle one." She certainly is that!

As significant and difficult was the choosing of our daughters' names, I cannot even imagine the task of naming each star in the universe. Yet, our God is so powerful and so wise, He did so!

The next time you look into a starry sky, take a moment to consider the wonder of God. As you reflect on His tender care for each star, try to imagine how special you are to Him!

APPLICATION:
1) If you do not already know it, research the meaning of your name.
2) What would you need to change in your life to live up to the meaning of your name?

PRAY and thank God for your name. Ask Him to help you live your life in such a way that your name will be synonymous with a godly reputation.

DEVOTIONAL FOR CHAPTER FOUR

Day Four

Scripture Reading: Psalm 30:1-12

Verse of the Day: . . . *weeping may remain for a night, but rejoicing comes in the morning* (Psalm 30:5).

We all have been there at one time or another. Our hearts are broken. We have disappointed someone, we have been disappointed by someone, or we have disappointed ourselves. We feel as if the fist of sorrow has such a hold around our hearts that it will squeeze the very life from what is left of the bruised tissue. We have cried so hard and long, we feel that no salty liquid is left in our bodies. The darkness of the night magnifies the darkness of our souls.

David knew the depth of such pain. Sadly, he lost sight not only of who he was, but also Who God was. He allowed lust to lead to adultery, deceit, and eventually murder. He, who had been a *man after* [God's] *own heart* (I Samuel 13:14), had become an enemy of the very nature of God.

Oscar Wilde once stated, "Where there is sorrow, there is holy ground." Truly, God is at work seeking to restore and renew broken hearts. David confessed his sin with godly sorrow. He repented of it. He sought restoration with God. He praised God for His loving forgiveness. He declared in Psalm 30:11, *"You turned my wailing into dancing; you removed my sackcloth and clothed me with joy."*

As the morning sky is brushed with the colorful strokes of dawn, we are reminded that it is indeed a new day. It is a day that has never been lived. It is time for the restoration of light, and the restoration of life. Truly, *weeping may remain for a night* but it is not night forever. Joy can and will *come in the morning* <u>and</u> "in the mourning!"

Step forward onto holy ground, and allow God to meet you. He is already there waiting for you.

Application:

1) What area(s) of your life is/are presently causing you pain?
2) Have you allowed God to work in them, or do you find security in hiding behind them?
3) Following David's example, allow God to heal your broken heart today.

PRAY and ask for the courage to face the things in your life that keep you living in the darkness of sorrow. Claim the joy that will *come in the morning!*

DEVOTIONAL FOR CHAPTER FOUR

Day Five

Scripture Reading: Matthew 24:5-42

Verse(s) of the Day: *Immediately after the distress of those days 'the sun will be darkened, and the moon will not give its light; the stars will fall from the sky, and the heavenly bodies will be shaken.' At that time the sign of the Son of Man will appear in the sky, and all the nations of the earth will mourn. . .* (Matthew 24:29,30).

Songs have been composed. Poems have been penned. Pictures have been painted. Books have been written. Dramas have been produced. Every avenue of expression has been used to depict the Second Coming of Jesus. Yet, as imaginative and descriptive as artists, authors, and actors have been, no mere human can comprehend how awesome and awe-inspiring that day will be.

Biblical prophecies foretell more about the Second Coming of Jesus than about His First Advent. Just as a great star accompanied His birth in Bethlehem (Matthew 2:2), today's focal passage relates that signs and wonders in the heavens will also accompany His Second Advent. The sun and moon will be darkened and the stars will fall from the heavens. Can we even begin to imagine what that will be like?

The events in Matthew 24 describe a time of great tribulation preceding Jesus' return to earth. In order of sequence, Jesus explained to His disciples what would transpire on the earth just prior to His appearance. This exposition was in response to their inquiry in v.3, "*. . . what will be the sign of your coming and of the end of the age?*"

As we look at the detailed list, we certainly are aware that the stage is being set for many of these events to take place. Jesus said, "*Therefore keep watch, because you do not know on what day your Lord will come*" (v.42).

For what are we to watch? We are to watch for the fulfillment of the events He described in Matthew 24. He clearly stated in v.33 that. *. . when you see all these things, you know that it is near, right at the door.* The question of eternal significance in life is "are you ready?" If the earth as we know it should end today, what will happen to you? When all is said and done, that is what really matters.

Songs, paintings, poems, books, dramas can lead our thinking in the direction of the Second Coming. However, nothing contrived by man can compare to that day when signs and wonders in the heavens will accompany the greatest day in the future of mankind.

Applicaton:
1) Examine your heart and life to see if you are ready for Jesus' return to earth.

PRAY for the wisdom and the courage to do what is necessary to prepare you for His return.

DEVOTIONAL FOR CHAPTER FOUR

Day Six

Scripture Reading: Ecclesiastes 3:1-11

Verse(s) of the Day: *There is a time for everything, and a season for every activity under heaven. . .* (Ecclesiastes 3:1).

He has made everything beautiful in its time. He has also set eternity in the hearts of men; yet they cannot fathom what God has done from beginning to end (Ecclesiastes 3:11).

Back to the Future was a box office hit produced in the 1980's. One thing that made the movie so popular with audiences was that every event occurring in the beginning of the movie was somehow repeated later in the movie, and then was resolved at the end. It was a fascinating journey from present life to future life then back to a somewhat altered present life.

Although the movie was fictional, it inspired the imaginations of those who viewed it. Moviegoers were left wondering what it would be like to experience life from the present to the future and back.

How many times have we wished we could see into the future and know how things will turn out in the end? In a real sense, we can! Although our future vision is limited because of the reality of the present, we do have certain promises and assurances in God's Word that allow us to glimpse into the future.

Today's focal passage is an example of this. The scripture is very clear that the things that happen in our lives are for a purpose: *There is a time for everything* (Ecclesiastes 3:1). Things happen in life for a purpose.

Though some situations may seem undesirable, when given to God they are used to bring about beauty in a person's life: *He has made everything beautiful in its time* (Ecclesiastes 3:11). God does the work. Our part is to remain patient while He is working and let Him take the time He needs to accomplish His purposes. The past, present, and future are in God's hands. Each season of life serves a purpose in making one's life the beautiful thing God intends for it to become.

Regrets from our past and worry about our future can cause us to miss the joy of the present season. On our refrigerator we display a clip from the comic strip "Family Circus" by Bill Keane. In it, the little sister is explaining to her younger brother that "Yesterday's the past, tomorrow's the future, but today is a GIFT. That's why it's called the PRESENT." Yes, each season is indeed a gift. Each season has its own beautiful purpose in life. . . *Back to the Future* and beyond!

Application:
1) Which season of your life do you have the most trouble giving to God? Is it your past, present, or future?
2) Ask God for the faith to trust Him in every season and circumstance of your life.

PRAY and ask God for the wisdom to accomplish His beautiful purposes in your life.

DEVOTIONAL FOR CHAPTER FOUR

Day Seven

Scripture Reading: Job 3:1-26

Verse of the Day: *God made two great lights—the greater light to govern the day and the lesser light to govern the night. He also made the stars* (Genesis 1:16).

Today's scripture reading is one of the most heart-wrenching passages in the Bible. The first chapter of Job sets the stage for the saga of a righteous man who loved God. Job was the wealthiest man in the east. He owned seven thousand sheep, three thousand camels, five hundred yoke of oxen, five hundred donkeys, a large house, many servants and he had a large family consisting of his wife, seven sons, and three daughters.

In a single day, Job lost everything he had, except his wife. A messenger reported that a band of thieves had stolen his oxen and donkeys and killed the servants attending them. While that messenger was still speaking, another came to inform him that fire had burned the sheep and the servants attending them. A third messenger came to report that three bands of thieves had stolen the camels and killed the servants attending them. A final messenger made it known that a great wind had struck the house of his oldest son, and all his children and servants had been killed.

Shortly thereafter, Job contracted a disease that covered his body with painful boils. In spite of all, Job did not curse God, but rather lamented the day he himself was born. Job felt the light of his life had been snuffed out by the darkness of his misery. Our problems often seem to overwhelm us in the dark of night.

A dear friend of mine, Teresa, recently experienced the death of her only child. For months we had anticipated her precious daughter giving birth. The day finally arrived. Complications arose. The baby lived, but Teresa's daughter died. The long awaited "due date" of the baby became the "death date" of Teresa's daughter. There simply are no words to express the darkness we experienced. There seemed to be perpetual darkness and night.

Recently Teresa asked, "Have you ever noticed that God gave only one light (the sun) for the day, but He gave two sources of light (the moon and stars) for the darkness of night?"

No, I had never noticed. I thank Teresa for pointing that out to me! God knew that in the darkness of night, you and I and all of mankind would need extra light.

God restored the light to Job. In the last chapter of the book of Job, we find that God blessed Job with twice as much material wealth as before, plus seven more sons, and three more daughters.

God is also restoring the light to Teresa. It happens each time she looks into the face of her grandson.

Application:

1) Are there certain problems that seem to overwhelm you during

the dark of night?
2) Identify them and determine not to dwell on them at night. Bring them to God's light.

PRAY and ask God to restore light to the dark areas of your life. He longs to do so!

CHAPTER FIVE

<u>BIBLICAL APPLICATION</u>

The Fifth Day of Creation

(Genesis 1:20-23)

20 And God said, "Let water teem with living creatures, and let birds fly above the earth across the expanse of the sky." 21 So God created the great creatures of the sea and every living and moving thing with which the water teems, according to their kinds, and every winged bird according to its kind. And God saw that it was good. 22 God blessed them and said, "Be fruitful and increase in number and fill the water in the seas, and let the birds increase on the earth." 23 And there was evening, and there was morning—the fifth day.

Heaven and earth were prepared for their respective inhabitants. Everything necessary to sustain animal life was now in place. God began the creation of the world on day one when He spoke light and happiness into existence. He separated the atmosphere from the waters on earth on the second day, summoned dry land and plant life on the third day, and suspended the sun, moon, and stars on the fourth day. God's light and happiness; air and water; land and edible plants; designations of time for activity and rest, seasons and religious observances, days and years were all in place for one of the most dramatic moments in history.

I. FISH

On the fifth day, God created the first animal life to dwell in His beautiful world. How carefully He had planned bountiful habitats, in which these living beings would reside and flourish! Now He was ready to take creation to a new level.

And God said. . . (Genesis 1:20) confirms that once again creation progressed with the spoken Word of God. The divine command of God produced the creatures brought into existence on this day. They did not just happen. They happened as part of the well-organized plan of the Almighty.

Let the water teem with living creatures. . . (Genesis 1:20). In this verse, the Hebrew word for "creatures" is *sherets* and it means "a swarm, for example, an active mass of minute animals." This is the only time in the Bible this particular word for "creature" is used, therefore it is unique to this day in the creation narrative. *Sherets* comes from the Hebrew word *sharats* which implies "to abound, to breed (bring forth, increase) abundantly."

The tiny aquatic animals, the first creations of animal life, were given a special ability to multiply and fill the waters of the earth. This was confirmed when, in Genesis 1:22, *God blessed them and said, "Be fruitful and increase in number and fill the waters in the seas. . ."* The Hebrew words for "fruitful" and "increase" are *parah* meaning "to grow, to increase" and *rabah* meaning "to increase in abundance, to be full of, to be more in number."

Creatures were the first creations in the Bible referred to as *living* (Genesis 1:20). Inherent in this phrase is the idea of "a living breath." This breath is what distinguishes the animal kingdom from the plant kingdom.

Certainly, plants are alive. Science confirms that they are living organisms whose functions in many ways resemble those of animals. Plants take in nutrients and give off waste, and they grow, reproduce, and eventually die.

However, one main characteristic that distinguishes animal life from plant life is the process of breathing, or respiration. Animals breathe in oxygen and give off carbon dioxide as a waste product. Although this happens on a smaller scale with plants, an opposite process dominates plant life.

During photosynthesis, plants take in carbon dioxide and give off oxygen. Amazingly, animals breathe in oxygen and give off carbon dioxide. Therefore, the "waste product" of each becomes the life-sustaining element of the other. God is so wise.

II. FOWL

God, continuing the command, spoke into existence *birds*. The Hebrew word for *birds* is *owph* meaning "a bird covered with feathers, or as a covering with wings."

These winged creatures were created to inhabit a particular place, to *fly above the earth across the expanse of the sky* (Genesis 1:20).

Thus were existing swarms of small aquatic creatures swimming in the waters of the earth, and flocks of winged creatures were flying in the heavens above the earth. The newly formed earth began teeming with animal life. To this very day fish and fowl continue to travel gregariously in schools and flocks as they did from the beginning of their creations.

Fish and Fowl

The narrative of the creative process of the fifth day continues: *So God created great creatures of the sea and every living and moving thing with which the water teems, according to their kinds. . . (Genesis 1:21).

From the swarms of small aquatic creatures to the great whales of the ocean, God, *Elohim*, created living beings. The word for *created* in this verse is the Hebrew word, *bara*, which indicates the making of something that is totally new. Only God can do that! We, as humans, can only create out of what already exists. We do not have the ability to actually "create," but merely to "re-create."

It is important to note that *bara* is the same word that is used in Genesis 1:1, *In the beginning God created the heavens and the earth.* Just as God created heaven and earth as a totally new thing, God also created animal life as a totally new thing. From the tiny aquatic creatures, to the great whales or "sea monsters," to the winged birds flying in the heavens, God created them through a divine act.

Likewise, . . . *every living and moving thing with which the water teems, according to their kinds. . . (Genesis 1:21) demonstrates that the Almighty created each individual species of marine life. In addition, *according to their kinds* points to the fact that each class was distinct when it was created and distinct when it obeyed God's command . . . *"Be fruitful and increase in number"*. . . (Genesis 1:22).

God continued the progression of creation with *every winged bird after its kind* (Genesis 1:21). Inherent in this seemingly generic phrase are all the distinct orders, species, and classes of the bird family. As with marine life, each grouping was created by God to be and to remain distinct within the animal kingdom.

The Blessing

Creations of the fifth day pleased their Creator. The closing phrase of Genesis 1:21 confirms that *God saw that it was good.* In fact, it was so good that *God blessed them and said, "Be fruitful and increase in number and fill the waters in the seas, and let birds increase on the earth"* (Genesis 1:22).

The Hebrew word used here for *bless* is *barak* meaning, "to kneel down as an act of adoration, to praise, to congratulate, to salute, to thank." The creations of the fifth day filled the Creator's heart with praise and thanksgiving.

God could see into the future, and He knew how vital His creations would be to the welfare of the creations that were to come. Specifically, His blessing upon them was that they would continue to fill His beautiful world with teeming life.

Not only were they to *be fruitful and increase in number* (Genesis 1:21) immediately after their creation, but infused into their nature was the capacity to constantly reproduce. They reproduce their own kind and they multiply in masses to this day.

And God saw that it was good (Genesis 1:21). Truly we can agree with God that the creations of the fifth day are good.

And there was evening, and there was morning—the fifth day. Have you ever noticed that we have a tendency to look at the beginning of a day in the morning as most important? God does the opposite. He looks at what we consider the ending, or evening, as the beginning. No matter how we start the day in the morning, how we finish by evening is what really counts. The evening began the fifth day of creation, the day that living beings were placed carefully within God's beautiful world.

NUTRITIONAL APPLICATION

The original diet in the Garden of Eden was that of the raw vegetables, seeds (including nuts, whole grains, and legumes), and fruits created on the third day. In Genesis 1:29 God told Adam and Eve, *"I give you every seed-bearing plant on the face of the whole earth and every tree that has fruit with seed in it. They will be yours for food."* Their diet of raw plant life was perfect in every way. It was given in the perfect environment to a physically perfect man and woman.

Originally, even the animals ate a plant-based, vegetarian diet. In Genesis 1:30 God said, *"'And to all the beasts of the earth and all the birds of the air and all the creatures that move on the ground—everything that has the breath of life in it—I give every green plant for food.' And it was so."*

During the Messianic age when Jesus will rule the "peaceable kingdom," scripture portrays that even animals which are presently carnivorous will return to the vegetarian diet first ordained for them. In Isaiah 11:7, which is a Messianic prophecy, it is written that *the cow will feed with the bear, their young will lie down together, and the lion will eat straw like the ox.* Also, in Isaiah 65:25, God assures that some day *the wolf and the lamb will feed together, and the lion will eat straw like the ox, but dust will be the serpent's food. They will neither harm nor destroy on all my holy mountain.*

The Flood

Adam and Eve were given the gift of free will, or the privilege of making choices. When they chose to yield to temptation and sin entered the world, each generation thereafter grew more abundantly sinful: *The Lord was grieved that he had made man on the earth, and his heart was filled with pain* (Genesis 6:6).

Genesis 6:5-9:29 records the biblical account of the universal flood and Noah's ark. According to Genesis 7:2, God instructed Noah to take seven couples (male and female) of "clean" animals and one couple of animals who were "not clean" into the ark. God also told him to take seven couples of birds on board in order to preserve their species.

This passage contains the first mention of "clean" and

"unclean" animals in the Bible. The Hebrew word for "clean" is *tahowr* meaning "to be bright; to be pure." In contrast, "not clean" in the biblical sense, later called "unclean," is *tame* meaning "foul, defiled, polluted."

How would Noah have known which animals were clean and unclean? Probably the concept already had been established from the time of Adam. When Adam's sons brought their offerings to God, Cain's produce was rejected and Abel's first-born lamb, a clean animal, was accepted. This was a beautiful foreshadowing of the Lamb of God, who one day would be the acceptable offering for the sins of the world.

In Genesis 6:20, God told Noah that the animals would come to him by pairs so that they could be kept alive. Later, in Genesis 7:1-2, God explained that seven pairs of clean animals and one pair of unclean animals would come to him, a supernatural event as God brought the animals to Noah. Since only clean animals were appropriate for sacrifices, it was important that he could distinguish between clean and unclean animals. The fact that God brought the appropriate animals to Noah clearly showed him, by the number of pairs that arrived, which were clean or unclean.

Generally speaking, the clean animals were more docile and able to be gathered for sacrifice. It appears that the unclean animals were on the ark only to preserve their species for proliferation after the flood. However, God in His providence was making ample provision for an abundance of the clean animals that would be used for both sacrificial and dietary purposes. In a real sense, all of this was a foreshadowing of the dietary laws that would be introduced to the nation of Israel at a later time.

The Introduction of Meat into the Diet

God's perfect plan given to Adam and Eve was that they enjoy bountifully the plant life created on the third day. As humans, our bodies are designed to excel on a plant-based diet. We have more teeth for crushing and grinding than we do for biting and tearing. Our jaws move from side to side for grinding as well as up and down for tearing and biting. Our saliva is alkaline more for the digestion of starch than animal protein. Our intestinal tracts are long allowing for the slow absorption of nutrients rather than short to rapidly expel the contents and rid the body of animal protein.

During the flood most of the vegetation on earth was destroyed. Therefore, after Noah and his family left the ark, God added another element to their diets as the earth's vegetation went through a process of re-growth.

The inclusion of meat in the diet of man is an example of God's permissible will. Although they were given permission to eat meat, they were still created to fare better on plant life than animal life. God did not change the design of their human bodies. His intention was never that mankind switch to the meat-based diet that dominates the Standard American Diet (SAD). Although consumption of animal flesh/products is permissible, it should be limited. Plant life should be our primary source of food.

In Genesis 9:2-4 God told Noah,

> *The fear and dread of you will fall upon all the beasts of the earth and all the birds of the air, upon every creature that moves along the ground, and upon all the fish of the sea; they are given into your hands. Everything that lives and moves will be food for you. Just as I gave you the green plants, I now give you everything. But you must not eat meat that has its lifeblood still in it.*

Originally man was given authority over the animals through Adam. God reminded Noah that he also had this control. It is possible that up until this time, animals had remained vegetarian eaters. (If any of them had been carnivorous, they could have devoured other animals while in the ark.) Now that meat was introduced into the diet, Noah may have feared that he and his small family would become prey to the animals that had been confined in the ark for so long.

God assured Noah that the animals would have a natural fear of him and his family. This assurance was not only for Noah, but for subsequent generations as well.

However, at this point, God did give one restriction regarding His permission to eat meat. Noah and his family were not allowed to eat any animal that had *its lifeblood still in it* (Genesis 9:4). The beginning chapter of <u>The Creation Diet</u> dealt with the fact from

Leviticus 17:14 that *the life of every creature is in its blood*.

This restriction was twofold in nature. The fact that no living animals could be consumed was God's protection against cruelty to animals. It was also a protection against Noah and his family consuming contaminated blood. A study conducted at Johns Hopkins University found that the blood of all animals that were tested was more toxic than their flesh. God protected mankind from this toxicity when he forbade eating the lifeblood of animals.

We are told in Genesis 8:20 that *Noah built an altar to the Lord and, taking some of all the clean animals and clean birds, he sacrificed burnt offerings on it*. What a bonfire that must have been! It is hard to imagine that many animals being sacrificed at one time.

It is not recorded that God put restrictions on which animals Noah could eat, but my logic leads me to reason that Noah ate only clean animals. Although he sacrificed some of each kind of clean animal, there would still be several pairs from the seven pairs of each left in existence for sacrifice and for food. However, if he had eaten the unclean animals, of which there was only one pair, none of their species would have been left to populate the earth.

I. FISH

Human beings could exist totally and healthfully on the creations of the first four days. That was God's perfect plan given to Adam and Eve. However, most people choose to eat meat deemed permissible after the flood. The Creation Diet reveals that the days of creation are listed according to what is most healthful for us. Therefore it is of little surprise that in the order of creation, fish were the first animals created.

Of all the meats available today, fresh fish are considered the healthiest choice. It is the meat whose protein is digested most easily by humans.

In Chapter Three of The Creation Diet we learned that nonessential fatty acids are produced by the body but essential fatty acids must come from the foods we eat. Most fish, especially fish that come from cold, deep waters, contain Omega-3 essential fatty acids. These cold-water fish are usually more fatty in the good sense that they contain more essential fatty acids than less fatty fish. Cold-water fish include salmon, sardines, anchovies, bluefish, herring, lake trout, mackerel, whitefish, and bluefin tuna. Primarily the essential fatty acids found in these fish are alpha-linolenic acid, eicosapentaenoic acid (EPA), and docosahexaenoic acid (DHA).

The omega-3 fatty acids in fish have been linked to lower levels of blood lipids, including triglycerides. In addition, they have been known to lower blood pressure. Recent studies conclude that even two meals a week of cold-water fish can reduce the risk of arrhythmia and sudden cardiac death. One reason is that omega-3 fatty acids serve as anti-clotting agents by reducing the ability of platelets to stick together, thinning the blood.

The omega-3 fatty acids also have anti-inflammatory properties that can help with pain prevention and control by blocking the formation of substances that trigger inflammation. This has also been found to help asthma. Even the prevention of migraine headaches has been associated with essential fatty acids found in fish.

Fish are naturally low in cholesterol and high in certain minerals, including selenium. The alkylglycerols found in the lipids of fish act as chelating agents, helping to remove heavy toxic metals from the body. In addition, fish oils help to curb the overproduction of prostaglandins in the body, thus reducing the risk of breast, pancreatic, lung, prostate, and colon cancers.

Psoriasis patients have responded well to treatment with omega-3 fish oils. In one startling study, a remarkable two-thirds of psoriasis patients improved quickly when they ingested the essential fatty acids found in fish.

As if all of this were not wonderful enough, DHA and tyrosine in fish also have been proven to increase the function of the brain. In fact, one study in Switzerland indicated that as little as two to three meals of fatty fish per week were significantly beneficial to the brain. The old saying that "fish feeds the brain" is partially true. Even though it does not actually feed the brain, it does improve its function.

In summary, fish and properties within fish have been known to do the following:

• Lower blood lipids, including triglycerides
• Lower blood pressure

- Reduce risk of heart disease
- Thin the blood
- Ease pain of inflammatory conditions such as arthritis
- Help prevent migraine headaches
- Clean the body from heavy toxic metals
- Relieve asthma
- Reduce the risk of some cancers
- Improve psoriasis
- Improve the function of the brain.

With this as evidence, we would do well to make fish our first choice of meat.

Jesus Ate Fish

Jesus is always the most perfect example we can follow. In the Bible there are several references to Jesus serving fish to others.

When He performed the miracle of feeding the five thousand, He multiplied and served *fish* and *barley loaves* (Matthew 14:17-21; Mark 6:30-44; John 6:1-15).

After the resurrection, Jesus provided a morning meal of grilled fish for His disciples: *When they landed, they saw a fire of burning coals there with fish on it, and some bread. . .* Jesus *said to them, "Come and have breakfast"* (John 21:9;12).

The only reference of Jesus actually eating fish was after the resurrection: *They gave him a piece of broiled fish, and he took it and ate it in their presence* (Luke 24:42,43).

The majority of disciples whom Jesus chose were fishermen. In fact, He used the analogy of fishing when referring to His disciples as evangelists-in-training: *"Come follow me," Jesus said, "and I will make you fishers of men"* (Matthew 4:19).

In His wisdom, God knew that His first created living beings would someday represent His blessed Son. During the persecution of the early church, the symbol of a fish was used as a secret sign among the believers, because the Greek word for fish is *ichthus*. The component Greek letters of "fish" became a sacred acrostic for "Jesus Christ, Son of God, Saviour." To this day, the sign of the fish is a symbol used among Christians.

Dietary Laws Concerning Fish and Marine Animals

The dietary laws of the Jews are of biblical origin and are found primarily in the books of Leviticus and Deuteronomy with a few references in Exodus. The dietary laws concern foods that should and should not be eaten, and how permissible foods must be prepared. The collection of Jewish dietary laws is known as *kashrut*, whose root word means "fit, proper, or correct." The commonly known word "kosher" comes from the same root.

Even though the dietary laws have health and hygienic benefits, the primary reason observant Jews keep the laws of *kashrut* is that they are commandments of God. It is as simple as that. God said it, so they observe it.

As previously mentioned, God told Noah to take seven pairs of "clean" animals and one pair of "not clean" or "unclean" animals on the ark. During the time of Moses, the understanding of clean and unclean animals was further expounded upon in the dietary laws in Leviticus 11:1-46 and Deuteronomy 14:4-21.

Many people have the opinion that clean and unclean animals, as well as the other dietary laws, are for Jewish people only. However, the nation of Israel did not originate until the time of Abraham, many centuries after God told Noah to take clean and unclean animals on the ark. Since Noah was not Jewish, it is evident that the idea of clean and unclean animals is important for all people to understand.

Peter's vision recorded in Acts 10:1-48 is often misunderstood among those of the Christian faith. It is actually a beautiful story of how the gospel should be taken by the early Jewish believers to the Gentiles. All the writers of the New Testament, except possibly Luke, were Jewish, and the first fifteen pastors of the church in Jerusalem were Jewish. It is believed that all the members of the early church were Jewish since there are no records of Gentile members until around ten years after Jesus' ascension. The entire structure of the early church was based on the structure of the synagogue. The Judeo-Christian faith is exactly that. It is the Christian faith rooted in Judaism.

Because Jesus was Jewish and the early church was Jewish, the disciples and church leaders had the misconception that to be a Christian you had to convert to Judaism. (Many of Paul's teachings dealt with this controversial subject.)

In Peter's vision, a sheet came down from heaven filled with a variety of animals, mostly those deemed unclean according to the *kashrut*. In his vision, Peter was told to kill and eat the animals. In horror, he responded that he could not for he had never eaten any unclean animal. A voice was then heard saying, *"Do not call anything impure that God has made clean"* (Acts 10:15).

Many have understood the phrase to mean that God deemed all meat as clean and that all kinds of animals could be eaten. However, Peter's vision was symbolic of *people* rather than *animals*. He responded to the leading of the Holy Spirit by going to the home of a Gentile named Cornelius.

Acts 10:28 records that, when Peter arrived at Cornelius' home, he said to the Gentiles who were assembled there, *"You are well aware that it is against our law for a Jew to associate with a Gentile or visit him. But God has shown me that I should not call any man impure or unclean."* Peter's vision was not about food, it was about people. His vision was not about abolishing the dietary laws of the Jews, rather it was about Jews extending to Gentiles the message of the death, burial, and resurrection of Jesus.

Later, the Jerusalem council met in response to the confusion concerning which Jewish laws should be observed by Gentiles in order to become a part of the Christian community. Some of the noteworthy people who attended that council were Paul, Barnabas, Peter, James, Silas, and Judas Barsabas. The beautiful account of this summit that changed the world is recorded in Acts 15:1-29.

The agreement among the council was that Gentiles were welcome to abide by the laws given in the Torah, but were not required to do so. (The 613 laws in the Torah are instructions on how to live a balanced life. In fact, the Hebrew word for "law," *torah*, means "a precept or a statute.") Gentiles were required only to do the following things recorded in Acts 15:29:

- Avoid eating food sacrificed to idols
- Avoid eating the blood of animals
- Avoid sexual immorality.

These requirements are based on God's covenant with Noah

after the flood, the sign of which was a rainbow. Originally there were three laws of Noah, also called Noachide Laws, that were expanded into seven "necessary things." In addition to the ones listed above, worship of the one true God, love for one's neighbor, avoidance of pagan rites, and avoidance of idolatry were also added.

It is amazing how modern research verifies the validity of the instructions found in the *kashrut*. When we realize how beneficial these precepts are, we will be more open to embrace rather than reject them. When we remove the part of "the law" that was completed by Jesus (such as the sacrificial system and the priesthood), what remains is a body of instructions that can benefit our relationship with God and our fellow man.

Clean and Unclean Fish and Marine Animals

The criterion for deeming an animal clean or unclean seems to be determined primarily by their source of food. Although specific marine animals are not mentioned as being clean or unclean, characteristics of edible ones are given. We find these portions of the *kashrut* in the following scriptures:

> *Of all the creatures living in the water of the seas and streams, you may eat any that have fins and scales. But all creatures in the seas or streams that do not have fins and scales—whether among all the swarming things or among all the other living creatures in the water—you are to detest. And since you are to detest them, you must not eat their meat and you must detest their carcasses. Anything living in the water that does not have fins and scales is to be detestable to you* (Leviticus 11:9-12).

> *Of all the creatures living in the water, you may eat any that has fins and scales. But anything that does not have fins and scales you may not eat; for you it is unclean* (Deuteronomy 14:9).

It is really quite simple. According to God's Word, marine life with fins and scales is clean and can be eaten. Marine life without fins and scales is unclean and cannot be eaten. Why is that so? What are the purposes of fins and scales? Fins are the paddle-like part of the fish that, when moved, allow the fish to swim swiftly through the water in search of the best sources of food. Scales are the hard, thin, flat plates that cover the skin of fish. They help protect the flesh of the fish from poisonous materials as they move through the water.

If a fish either lacks scales, or has a different type of scale, it is considered unclean. Many people are dismayed to learn that all types of shellfish and bottom-dwellers lack both fins and scales. This includes the crustacean group of shellfish consisting of shrimp, crab, lobster, crayfish, and barnacles. It also includes other shellfish such as scallops, oysters, mussels, and clams. In addition, turtles, frogs, and snails are considered unclean. These animals do not possess fins enabling them to move swiftly through the water in search of food, nor the filtering system provided by scales.

A common characteristic of the above named scale-less and fin-less animals is that they are known as scavengers. They eat whatever happens to be in the environment around them. Many of them, such as oysters, lie in beds waiting to ingest whatever comes their way.

If shellfish are placed in bodies of water laden with sewage, chemicals, parasites, viruses, and bacteria, they actually will purify the water by eating the contaminants. As they ingest these harmful substances, their flesh becomes contaminated by the disease-causing organisms. In addition, shellfish have a tendency to carry heavy concentrations of metals in their flesh. Two metals most often found in the flesh of shellfish are mercury and lead.

Several years ago, the state Legislature in California proposed a law that would require the food industry to label all shellfish, "This food may be hazardous to your health." Is it any wonder God's Word says that we should not eat these foods?

The following is a list of clean and unclean sea animals and fish to aid in making the wisest selections:

Clean and Unclean Marine Life

CLEAN *(with fins and scales)*	UNCLEAN *(without fins and scales)*
Anchovy	Billfish
Barracuda	Catfish
Black bass	Cutlassfish
Black drum	Eel
Bluefish	Firefish
Bonito	Gar
Carp	Goosefish
Channel Bass	Lamprey
Chub	Leatherjacket
Cod	Lomosucker
Croaker	Marlin
Flounder	Ocean Pout
Flying Fish	Octopus
Goldfish	Oilfish
Grouper	Puffer
Haddock	Rock Prickleback
Hake	Sailfish
Halibut	Sand Skate
Herring	Sculpin
Kingfish	Shark*
Mackerel (except Snake Mackerel)	Snake Mackerel
Mahimahi	Stingray
Mullet	Sturgeon*
Orange Roughy	Swordfish *
Perch	Toadfish
Pike	Triggerfish
Pollock	Trunkfish
Pompano	Wolfish
Porgy	(Whales, Dolphins
Rainbow Trout	and Porpoises are
Rock Bass	mammals. Since
Rockfish	they do not meet
Salmon	the criteria for
Sardine	clean mammals, they
Sea Bass	are considered
Shad	unclean.)
Smelt	
Sole	Shellfish:
Spanish Mackerel	Clams
Spot	Conch
Trout	Crabs
Tuna (bluefin)	Crayfish
Walleye	Lobster
Whitefish	Mussels
Whiting	Oysters
	Scallops
	Shrimp

Due to their unusual scales, Jewish law does not allow these.

CHOICES THAT DIMINISH THE BENEFITS OF FISH

Clean vs. Unclean

The most obvious way to destroy the benefits of God's first living creations is to choose to eat the ones that are not healthful. Eating unclean, scavenger types of animals can cause toxic conditions in our bodies. God promises special blessings to those who obey His instructions. However, as with all choices in life, each person must decide what he or she will do in this matter.

Reproductive Cloning

Because reproductive cloning has the potential of producing severe genetic disorders and defects, all cloned animals and products from cloned animals should be avoided. The extent of hazard to human health has not yet been determined.

Processing

Unfortunately, chemical preservatives are added to fresh fish to give them a longer shelf life. If buying in a grocery store, check the label to see if anything has been added to the fish.

Fresh fish are processed often for the convenience of quick meals. Fish are breaded with a heavy batter, precooked, and frozen. Again, check the ingredients' label to see what has been added during processing.

Poor Choices When Shopping

When shopping for fish, if at all possible, identify the source from which it was caught. Make every effort to refrain from buying fish from polluted waters. In an article, "Animal Waste Pollution in America: An Emerging Problem," Senator Tom Harkin stated that from 1995 to 1997 over 11 million fish died as a result of animal waste being dumped into the waterways of America. This animal waste came mainly from poultry and pig farms.

In addition to animal waste, man-made chemical waste is also polluting our fresh water supplies. The many types of chlorinated hydrocarbon pesticides are extremely stable compounds that do not break down easily, staying active for decades. According to some researchers, they can even exist for centuries.

Unfortunately, fish absorb chemicals through swimming and breathing in contaminated waters. They accumulate the pollutants inside their bodies, and this is passed on to those who ingest their flesh. The best choice is fresh fish that come from cold, deep waters far from polluted coastlines. Cold water fish are also the ones that contain the higher amounts of essential fatty acids.

If you are selecting fresh fish, look for the following clues:

1) Fish should not smell fishy. A fishy smell indicates that the fish are not fresh.
2) The flesh of the fish should be firm and not covered with anything.
3) If you are buying a whole fish, check the eyes to see if they are firm and clear.
4) If you are purchasing processed rather than fresh fish, check to see that no preservatives have been added for longer shelf life. Also, frozen is preferred over canned because the high heat used in canning changes the molecular structures of fish.

Methods of Cooking

Many times the benefits of nutritious foods are destroyed by the ways they are prepared. Frying or deep-frying is not the most healthful way to cook fish. When fish is fried it usually is dipped in a thick breading batter, or at the very least, white processed flour.

Fish should be cooked at moderate rather than high temperatures. Cooking at high temperatures not only dries out the fish, it results in the loss of healthful juices.

Baking, broiling, grilling, or poaching fish are the best choices of preparation. When broiling fish, cook it at least six inches from the broiler, and if grilling, six inches from the fire.

When dining out, ask that fish be prepared in one of these ways. However, if you are ordering fish and it only comes fried, remove as much of the breading as possible.

II. FOWL

The second class of living beings created by God is also the second most healthful type of meat, if eaten in an unadulterated state. Isn't God amazing?

The fowl created, as referred to in Genesis 1:20, in their natural states, contain elements that are quite healthy for mankind. Although fish is the healthiest of all meats, there are also benefits to eating poultry and the eggs of poultry.

In living cells enzymes change certain oils into substances called prostaglandins. It has been found that prostaglandins in pure chicken have strong antiviral properties. The old wives' tale that "Chicken soup is good for what ails you" could be more fact than fiction.

Tryptophan found in poultry, particularly turkey, has a calming effect on the body. Have you ever noticed that you are sleepy after eating the typical Thanksgiving dinner?

The protein in chicken and other fowl is fairly easy to digest. The easiest protein to digest is from plants, the next from fish, and thirdly from fowl, the same order in which God created them!

However, the fat content in poultry is higher than most people realize. Skinless roasted light meat derives about 18% of its calories from fat, and skinless roasted dark meat is 32% fat. Another surprising fact is that chicken is comparable to beef in its cholesterol content, each containing about 25 milligrams per 3 ounces.

With all of this taken into consideration, even poultry consumption should be limited. One suggestion is to use it more often as a condiment in casseroles and vegetable dishes than as the focal point of the meal.

Eggs

Pure eggs, mentioned in various places in the Bible, are good sources of protein. They contain the nutrients choline and inositol which are good for the central nervous system, the liver, and the gallbladder.

It is true that eggs contain an abundance of cholesterol. However, they also contain the nutrient lecithin which aids in the utilization of the cholesterol.

In addition, eggs contain all the amino acids needed by the body, as well as many vitamins and minerals. However, even as wonderful as they sound, we should limit the amount we consume. A good rule of thumb is one egg per day including what we eat in cooked foods. Both white and brown eggs have the same nutritional value.

Clean and Unclean Fowl

Unlike the clean and unclean fish in the Bible, no characteristics of fowl are listed. Instead, a detailed list of unclean fowl is found in Deuteronomy 14:11-18.

> *You may eat any clean bird. But these you may not eat: the eagle, the vulture, the black vulture, the red kite, the black kite, any kind of falcon, any kind of raven, the horned owl, the screech owl, the gull, any kind of hawk, the little owl, the great owl, the white owl, the desert owl, the osprey, the cormorant, the stork, any kind of heron, the hoopoe, and the bat.*

As with the unclean fish, the birds on the forbidden list are scavengers. Inherent in this passage is the fact that if a particular fowl is not on the list of unclean birds, it is permissible to eat them. However, in the United States market, the only poultry on the "kosher" market today are chicken, turkey, duck, and goose.

CHOICES THAT DIMINISH THE BENEFITS OF FOWL

Adulteration of Poultry Food

Originally, God designed poultry (the fowl most consumed in America) to hunt, root, scratch, and find the foods they needed. They roamed in open spaces and were very much in tune to the environment in which they lived.

Sadly, the poultry that consumers eat today are vastly different from farm-raised poultry of 30 years ago. Approximately 98% of the poultry and eggs in America come from "chicken farms," which are more like factories than farms. It is not unusual to find 80,000 or more chickens being raised on poultry farms.

In the case of laying chickens, on the average, five of them are confined to a cage measuring 16 inches by 18 inches. On some farms, the cages are as small as 12 inches by 12 inches. The cages with wire mesh "floors" are stacked floor to ceiling in large buildings without windows or proper ventilation.

The animals are fed a diet that is not only unhealthy for the poultry, but also unhealthy for the consumers who eat them. Prices are determined by weight, so the manufacturers put emphasis on producing heavy poultry. Poultry food on these modern-day farms is often made of combinations of the following: grain; overabundance of soy beans (to increase the protein in order to "fatten up" the poultry); stale discarded bakery goods; restaurant grease; fish-meal; and "animal protein" including parts of diseased animals that were condemned in the slaughterhouses.

In addition, the feed is laced with antibiotics due to high incidences of infections among the animals. From the time these animals are born, their antibiotic-laced diets are totally foreign to foods they would find in nature. Sulfur drugs, antibiotics, vaccines and even compounds of arsenic are fed consistently to the poultry we consume.

These toxins become stored in the flesh of the animals. Over a period of time, the poultry build up a resistance to the antibiotics and disease develops. When we as humans ingest the antibiotics stored in the flesh of animals, we begin to develop resistance to these antibiotics as well.

Foodborne Illnesses
It stands to reason that if we eat poultry that are diseased, disease can be transmitted to us. Most people tend to think only of Salmonella in conjunction with poultry. However, there are nine major foodborne pathogens, eight bacteria, and one parasite, that cause human illnesses in the United States. Of the nine, poultry are a major source of approximately 2/3 of them.

In a recent study, <u>Consumer Reports</u> found that harmful bacteria were present in 71% of the chickens bought in stores. One startling government report cited that over 90% of the chickens tested had lukeosis, which is chicken cancer.

Currently a bird flu strain has swept poultry populations around the world resulting in the deaths of hundreds of thousands of birds. Health officials fear that the virus may mutate into one that could be transmitted to humans causing a global epidemic.

Irradiation of Eggs
The irradiation of eggs is now a practice in the United States. Eggs are exposed to varying levels of radiation both to reduce food-

borne disease (by killing microorganisms considered to be harmful) and to extend shelf life.

Irradiation changes the flavor and texture of the eggs. Yolks are more watery and have less color than normal eggs. The irradiation process also destroys vitamins, minerals, and other nutrients in foods. A major concern is that it can lead to the formation of free radicals in the bodies of those who ingest irradiated foods. There is also suspicion that this could lead to mutant forms of the very bacteria scientists are hoping to kill by the procedure.

Processing

Most consumers are not aware of the various aspects of poultry processing. A general description is as follows:

Poultry are grabbed, usually at night, either manually by people called "stuffers" or by an automated machine called a "poultry harvester."

The poultry are then crowded into crates (in the case of chickens around ten to twelve per crate), stacked on top of each other, and transported to slaughterhouses.

The birds wait in the truck until their turn to be processed. Sometimes the animals do not survive the temperatures as they are waiting on the truck.

The killing of poultry usually involves the following three phases:

1) The birds are hung upside down by the feet and dragged through a 12-foot trough filled with electrified water to which salt has been added (to improve conduction). This "stunning" is meant to relax the birds and render them unconscious for the slaughter. However, as many birds are struggling during this time, they often miss the stun bath.
2) The necks of the birds are cut by blades either manually or mechanically. Then they are automatically conveyed to the bleed-out tunnel where blood drains from their bodies. Often post-slaughter stunning is performed for large birds that may be alive still. This process involves the poultry being guided automatically against an electrified ladder or plate.

3) The poultry are dipped into a scalding bath to remove the feathers. Afterwards, they are processed for their intended purposes such as whole birds, poultry parts, or animal feed. Often this processing means the addition of chemicals used as preservatives for longer shelf life.

It is estimated that more than 25 million poultry animals are processed every day in the United States. Given the mass numbers that constantly are going through the above named processing procedures, consumers have cause to be concerned about hygienic standards.

In the past, government inspectors have condemned poultry considered "unwholesome," meaning those that exhibited such things as parasites, tumors, sores, and disease. At the present time, newly released standards no longer allow governmental officials to inspect each carcass in order to approve its wholesomeness. That responsibility has been turned over to plant officials. Government inspectors now make overall evaluations of the plants' performances in general. They sample a portion of the plant production during various shifts to determine if company employees are removing a sufficient amount of unwholesomeness from the poultry.

Before ending this section, it is important to say a word about the more humane process of slaughtering animals according to the *kashrut*, which also ensures more safety for the consumer. A very specific way of slaughter, called *shechitah*, is required according to Jewish dietary law, and only can be administered by a trained ritual slayer, known as a *shochet*. When properly done, this kosher method assures a minimal amount of suffering for the animals.

A perfectly sharpened blade, free from even the slightest nick or unevenness, is used. The knife moves swiftly over the wind and food pipes in a fraction of a second, severing the trachea, esophagus, the two vagus nerves, both carotid arteries, and the jugular veins. Research has shown that, when done properly, this method of slaughter results in the instant loss of consciousness. There appears to be no pain during the fraction of a second before unconsciousness. The lack of pain in this procedure has been compared to the fact that when you cut yourself shaving with a sharp razor, you do not feel pain for a split second until blood appears. Likewise, when done properly, animals are unconscious before pain could be felt.

Poor Choices When Shopping

The bottom line of poultry farms, as with most big businesses, is to make money. The practices they employ are to keep the cost down so consumers are able to buy more products.

There are places where poultry are raised in conditions closer to their natural habitats other than what poultry farms provide. However, the cost increases when the poultry are raised and processed in more favorable conditions. The question becomes, "What are we willing to pay for our health and the humane treatment of the animals we consume?"

If we determine that we are willing to pay more for healthful choices, a logical inquiry is, "Where can I find poultry that is raised in a natural environment, not polluted with chemical toxins, not diseased, and carefully processed?" This is not an easy question, but it is one for which there are answers worth seeking.

Of course, buying meats and eggs from a local farmer who raises poultry the "old-fashioned" way is a viable possibility. However, if this is not a feasible option, there are other alternatives.

Detective work is necessary to find healthy sources. Find suppliers of poultry at health food stores, and contact the sources to inquire about the raising and processing of their poultry. Specifically you want to seek sources that do the following:

- Allow poultry to be "free range" (also called "free roaming") rather than confined to battery cages.
- Provide poultry with proper ventilation and lighting when inside the poultry houses.
- Raise chemical-free poultry and eggs.
- Ensure that humane practices are used in the slaughtering, and that chemicals are not used in the processing.

According to the Food Safety and Inspection Service of the United States Department of Agriculture, "free range" or "free roaming" on labels mean that the poultry have been allowed outside. "Fresh" poultry are stored at a temperature no lower than 26° Fahrenheit and "frozen" at 0° EF (below Celsius) or below.

"Natural" poultry contain no artificial flavoring, coloring, or chemical preservatives, and they have been minimally processed, meaning the raw product has not been altered. Each "natural" label should explain what is included in the term.

Across America there is a phenomenon developing which addresses this problem in a helpful way. Individuals and families are forming co-op groups. Once a good source for healthy poultry and eggs is found, orders are placed directly with the farm or processor and then shipped to one location, and the co-op members (or someone hired by them) divide and distribute the food to those who ordered it. This requires a lot of work, but cuts down on cost significantly. A minimal number of participants, usually around fifteen, is required to form a co-op.

Also, there are a few grocery stores that have services available for placing special orders if enough people request that they do so. It would be worthwhile to check with your local grocer to determine the possibilities.

Methods of Cooking

Because of the high incidence of food-borne pathogens in poultry, it is very important to carefully prepare the meat for cooking. Poultry should be washed thoroughly, and any surface exposed to the meat or its juices should be cleaned and disinfected.

Remember that approximately half of the calorie content in chicken is in the skin. Therefore, skinning the chicken is more healthful than eating chicken with skin.

As with all proteins from animal sources, poultry (and eggs) should be cooked on moderate to low heat. If grilling, keep at least six inches away from the source of heat. It is very important to make sure that poultry are cooked completely before eating.

SPIRITUAL APPLICATION

Respect for Animal Life

God created the world with love and care. Each element of creation is dear to God's heart. The animals created on the fifth day were the first living beings brought into existence by the Almighty.

As seen in Genesis 1:22, *God blessed them and said, "Be fruitful and increase in number and fill the water in the seas."* As cited earlier in this chapter, the Hebrew word used for *bless* is *barak*. This special word means "to kneel down as an act of adoration; to praise; to congratulate; to salute; to thank."

The Creator Himself adored, praised, congratulated, saluted, and thanked the fish and fowl for their significance to His wonderful world. As will be seen in the next chapter, man was later given dominion over the animals. They were to be in subjugation to him. However, they were to be cared for by man even as God cared for each creation of life.

I cannot end this chapter without pointing out how animals are treated in the modern day meat industry. Webster defines "humane" as "kind; merciful; not cruel or brutal." The word "inhumane" means the opposite, "lacking compassion or kindness." The meat industry in America has become an inhumane institution, and the blame does not fall on any one person or group. We as consumers have demanded abundant supplies and low prices. In response to our demands, the industry "produces" animals like commodities rather than living beings carefully created and blessed by God.

Often the bodies of fish are pulverized during vacuum fishing. Many times they are gutted while their hearts still are beating.

Equally inhumane is how poultry are mistreated. The practices of the modern poultry industry have taken away the very things that make this species distinctive.

One of these distinctions is that poultry are sociable animals, establishing a hierarchy within the flock of up to ninety. They know each animal in the flock and they recognize their place in the hierarchy, hence the term "pecking order."

They also are very much in tune with nature. They tend to sleep in huddles at night, and rise early. Anyone who has ever been awakened by the crow of a rooster at daybreak knows this to be true. In addition, it is their nature to scratch, root, and seek food.

Several practices that rob poultry of their distinctive qualities are as follows:

- **Crowded, unnatural living conditions**
  Poultry are crammed into warehouses with artificial lighting

and conditions foreign to their natural instincts. Chickens, which lead the numbers of processed poultry, are divided into two categories: "broilers" and "layers." Broilers are raised for meat, and layers for egg production.

Broilers live in crowded warehouses with many thousands of birds standing or sitting in one place in the warehouse. The littered floor on which they live is filled with chicken feces and ammonia from urine.

Layers are crowded into wire cages stacked floor to ceiling. The average number of chickens in a laying warehouse is 80,000. Artificial lighting in these warehouses is manipulated to confuse the chickens. At birth they are left in total darkness except during feeding times. Then, as they begin to lay, they are exposed to artificial lighting almost continuously (seventeen hours or more each day). This is done to encourage the laying of eggs by the hens.

Urine and feces from the chickens on the top rows flow down through the wire cages to the chickens in the bottom cages, creating a breeding ground for infection and disease.

Their feet become entangled in the wire floor cage, so many chicken farmers amputate the toes of the chickens as a means of prevention. This is a very painful procedure for the animals.

Also, because of the crowded conditions, frustration prompts the birds to peck each other, resulting in the development of open sores and lesions. In an attempt to prevent this, another atrocity has been developed.

- **Debeaking**
Poultry beaks are extracted with a hot machine blade. The tissue around the beak is especially sensitive. In fact, it is compared to the skin underneath the fingernail of a human. Research shows that the disfigured birds often suffer lifelong pain as a result of debeaking. Many die because they no longer are able to eat food or drink water.

- **Forced Rapid Growth**
Poultry meat is priced according to weight, so most poultry farmers try to manipulate the growth of their animals. Poultry food is laced with ingredients that will cause them to grow rapidly, and the skeletal structure of poultry is not designed to handle this excess

weight. As a result, most of the birds are doomed to a lifetime of chronic pain and various disorders including fractures and joint dislocations.

- **Forced Molting**

  When layers slow their production of eggs, forced molting is used to increase production. Fluorescent lighting, which previously has been left on for seventeen hours or more hours daily, is removed. Simultaneously, as the hens are thrust into complete darkness, food and water are also removed. After a few days, water is reintroduced to the birds. Then light and food are returned, trying to make the hens feel that things have returned to "normal." This return to "normalcy" causes them to begin producing eggs again.

- **Elimination of male chicks**

  Since male chicks are of no use in the manufacture of eggs, they are usually disposed of quickly. In the hatcheries, male chickens are weeded from the trays and thrown into heavy plastic bags where they are suffocated. Every day in America approximately half a million baby chickens are disposed of in this way.

Who is to blame for these atrocities? Is it the consumer? Is it the farmer? Is it the processor? Is it the government? Or, is it all of us?

God *blessed* the animals He created on the fifth day. Do we?

Dear God,

Please forgive me. Forgive me when I allow convenience to supercede what is right. Thank You for creating the fish and the fowl. Our world would be so empty without them and You knew that. Thank You for blessing them. Help me to do my part each day to ensure that my world is more humane than it would have been had I not lived. Help me to become a part of the solution and not the problem.

In Jesus' name I pray, Amen.

MEMORY VERSE FOR CHAPTER FIVE:

Of all the creatures living in the water of the seas and the streams, you may eat any that have fins and scales (Leviticus 11:9).

ASSIGNMENT(S) FOR CHAPTER FIVE:

1) **Seek healthful sources** of fish and poultry.

2) Limit intake to **1 to 1 ½ servings (3-4 oz.) daily** of "clean" fish or "clean" fowl. This amounts to a serving approximately the size of a deck of cards.

3) Consumption of fresh eggs from "free range" chickens should be limited to **one egg daily, including those in cooked foods.**

DEVOTIONAL FOR CHAPTER FIVE

Day One

Scripture Reading: Jonah 1:1-17; 2:10

Verse of the Day: *But the Lord provided a great fish to swallow Jonah, and Jonah was inside the fish three days and three nights* (Jonah 1:17).

Have you ever noticed that God will use any means He deems necessary to accomplish His purposes? Who would have thought that a rebellious prophet would end up in the belly of a big fish? Yet today's featured verse clearly states that God had *provided* the fish for that purpose.

God told Jonah, a Jewish prophet, to go to Nineveh to preach the message of repentance. Jonah had no desire to go to this well-known city in Assyria. The cruelty of the Assyrians was unparalleled in ancient history. Some of their torturous practices included pulling out the tongues of their victims by the roots, flaying the skin of war prisoners inch by inch to stretch their skins on the city walls, and impaling people on long poles and raising them into the air until they died. It has been said that large piles of human heads marked the path of these brutal conquerors. Can you imagine how difficult it must have been for Jonah to consider taking a message of repentance to such people?

In fact, we are told in today's scripture passage that *Jonah ran away from the Lord and headed for Tarshish* (Jonah 1:3). However, the real heart of the matter is mentioned twice in this same verse. Jonah was trying to flee from God.

How clearly the love and mercy of God are demonstrated in this short book of the Bible! As cruel, wicked, and godless as the people of Nineveh were, Almighty God still loved them and longed for them to come into a relationship with Him.

The real miracle of this story is not that Jonah lived after being swallowed by a great fish. There have been several documented accounts of the same thing happening to other people. The real miracle is that just as God had not given up on the people of Nineveh, He also had not given up on Jonah. God gave him a second chance. When the fish deposited Jonah onto dry land, . . . *the word of the Lord came to Jonah a second time: "Go to the great city of Nineveh and proclaim to it the message I give you"* (Jonah 3:1).

This time Jonah went where God told him to go and did what God told him to do. What was the result? The answer is found in Jonah 3:5 when *the Ninevites believed God. They declared a fast, and all of them, from the greatest to the least, put on sackcloth.* God not only had provided a great fish to accomplish His purpose, but He also had prepared a great prophet!

<u>Application</u>:
1) Are you trying to run from the presence of God?
2) What do you think will happen if you surrender to His leading? What do you think will happen if you do not?

PRAY and ask God to help you develop a heart that is willing to obey Him.

DEVOTIONAL FOR CHAPTER FIVE

Day Two

Scripture Reading: Deuteronomy 6:4-9

Verse of the Day: *Which of you, if his son asks for bread, will give him a stone? Or if he asks for a fish, will give him a snake?* (Matthew 7:9,10)

Today's scripture reading begins with a passage which, in Hebrew, is known as the *Shema*. The word *shema* means "hear." God longs that we hear the important message that He is the one true God. He commands that this truth be passed down from father to child throughout all generations.

In Matthew 7:9,10, Jesus used a form of exaggeration to show that fathers (and mothers) desire to meet the needs of their children. The greatest need that any child has, or will ever have, is for someone to take the time to teach him or her about God. *Shema!*

One of the saddest stories I have ever heard is, unfortunately, true. A young boy, who had an extremely busy father, longed for the day his father would take him fishing. He was an obedient child who did not ask for much, but his heart's desire was to go fishing with his dad. Each time he asked, the answer was always the same, "Not today, Son, I have to work."

Finally, one beautiful morning his father awakened him and instructed him to hurry and dress because they were going fishing. It was the happiest day of the boy's childhood, for he had his father all to himself the entire day.

Years passed, and the boy grew into a man. As he left home to pursue his career, the memory of that glorious day, fishing with his father, was indelibly etched in his mind.

Some time later, his father died. As he and his mother were sorting through his father's belongings, he discovered that his father had kept daily journals. With shaky hands he nervously searched to find the journal entry for the day he and his dad had gone fishing. He was anxious to see how his father had described what he himself had considered the happiest day of his life.

He found the year, the month, and eagerly thumbed to the day. There it was! His heart pounded as he began to read. That day's entry was short, stating, "Did not go to the office today. Did not get any work done. Went fishing with my son. Day wasted."

The old saying, "The best things in life are free" is true. A day fishing and talking about the things of God would cost nothing except time. And it could end up being the happiest day of someone's life...maybe yours!

Application:

1) Think back to what you consider to be the happiest time of your childhood.
2) With that in mind, determine to live each day making memories and not regrets.

PRAY for God's help with setting priorities of time for yourself and those you love.

DEVOTIONAL FOR CHAPTER FIVE

Day Three

Scripture Reading: Luke 5:1-11

Verse of the Day: . . . *Put out into deep water, and let down the nets for a catch* (Luke 5:4).

They had worked all night and had caught not a single fish. They were tired. In fact, they already were washing their nets, ready to quit for a while. Can you imagine how exasperated Peter must have been when Jesus told him to *put out into deep water* again? I must admit that I am proud of Peter and crew. Although they probably thought it was useless, they went back out to sea and let down their nets in complete obedience to the words of Jesus.

Notice that as soon as they fully obeyed, they were blessed beyond their wildest imaginations. *When they had done so* (Luke 5:6a), the nets became so full they began to break, and back-up help had to be summoned. Then both boats almost sank because they were so full of fish.

It all began with obedience to the command, *"Put out into deep water."* In order to receive the blessings, we must be willing to get back in the boat. No matter how tired we may be. No matter how many times we have tried and failed. No matter how badly we want to quit. As long as He summons us to a task, we must climb back on board and move forward.

The obedience of the disciples resulted in the following:

- The occurrence of a spiritual renewal (v.8)
- Everyone around was astonished by what happened (v.9)
- They were promised even greater miracles (v.10)
- They left everything and followed Him (v.11)

These hard-working fishermen had learned one of the greatest lessons of life. Blessings come through obedience and partial obedience is no obedience at all. To experience the blessings of obedience we must *put out into deep water*. When we do, our blessings will be more than we ourselves can contain. We will have to share them with others!

Application:

1) Is there something in your life God is calling you to do, but you are afraid to "get back in the boat?"
2) What do you think will happen if you do?
3) What do you think will happen if you do not?

PRAY and ask God for the willingness to be obedient, even if it means leaving the security of the shore and putting out into the deep.

DEVOTIONAL FOR CHAPTER FIVE

Day Four

Scripture Reading: Song of Songs (Song of Solomon) 2:1-12

Verse of the Day: *Flowers appear on the earth; the season of singing has come, the cooing of doves is heard in our land* (Song of Songs 2:12).

Many people have questioned why Song of Songs was included in the canonization of the Bible. Some people see it merely as a sensual story of King Solomon and a Shulamite girl. In fact, in the Jewish tradition it was forbidden to read some portions of this book until the age of thirty.

However, Song of Songs is more than an earthly love story. This can be seen through the meanings of many of the phrases in the Hebrew context. To the Jewish person, this book represents the love between God and the nation of Israel. To the Christian, it represents the love between Jesus and His Bride, the Church.

One thing is seen clearly in this short book of the Bible. A progression of love is painted beautifully with words. In today's passage, "first love" is developing to a deeper level. It is a picture of our maturing relationship with Christ.

In Israel, there are basically two seasons, winter and summer. In winter, late September to March, it rains frequently and is quite dreary. Winter is often associated with bondage. Summer, on the other hand, is bright and sunny. This passage proclaims that the oppression of winter has passed and the beauty and freedom of summer have come.

Jesus, our Bridegroom, has released us from the shackles of sin. For those who have accepted His love and have chosen to become His Bride, . . . *the season of singing has come, the cooing of doves is heard in our land* (Song of Songs 2:12b).

We would do well to take some lessons from birds. Life is not always easy for them. They have to face incredible hardships in their flights of life. Yet no matter what, they are faithful to sing. The Hebrew words that are used in this verse mean more than merely the singing of the birds. The original language implies that it is a time for singing for all. Throughout scripture, singing is equated with praising God. This verse seems to express, "It is time for every living being to sing God's praises!"

Life has been described as a series of seasons. Which season are you in at this time? Have you responded to the love of the

Bridegroom, and passed from winter into summer? Or are you still in the dreariness of winter, so close, yet so far from the brightness of summer? The birds **are** singing. Do you hear them? Even more importantly, are **you** singing with them? The time of the singing has come.

Application:
1) In which season have you spent most of your life? Why?
2) What do you think it would take to "keep the birds singing" in your life?

PRAY and ask God to help you grow and mature in your love for the Bridegroom. Ask Him to help you make "the singing of praises" a part of every season of your life.

DEVOTIONAL FOR CHAPTER FIVE

Day Five

Scripture Reading: Isaiah 40:21-31

Verse of the Day: *Even youths grow tired and weary, and young men stumble and fall; but those who hope in the Lord will renew their strength. They will soar on wings like eagles; they will run and not grow weary, they will walk and not be faint* (Isaiah 40:30,31).

My father-in-law was a gentle, kind man from the hills of Tennessee. He amused us with some of the funniest witticisms I have ever heard. One of them was, "It seems like all people ever do any more is hurry up and wait."

As amusing as that statement is, it is also very true. We live in a world where we do not want to wait for anything. We are always in a hurry. We have fast foods, fast cars, fast computers, and we push our children to grow up too fast. We get impatient waiting for stoplights, checkout lines, appointments, and the end of worship services.

Yet in the midst of all this hurrying, aided by conveniences that are designed to save us time, we seem to be more tired and stressed than ever. Even our children and young people are weary from this fast-paced lifestyle.

This beautiful verse of the day offers hope. In the King James Version of the Bible, the phrase *hope in the Lord* is translated *wait upon the Lord*. As hard as that may seem, it is the only way we will find peace in life. God promises that if we wait on Him, we will *soar on wings like eagles*.

That is not just a random thought. Several good reasons explain why Isaiah used this phrase. Eagles are noted for their power and strength. They also are known for their ability to *mount up* and soar. In fact, their long, broad wings were designed for soaring. The wingspan of an eagle is between 72 to 90 inches. For eagles, soaring requires very little wing flapping.

Eagles have about 7,000 feathers that are lightweight, but very strong. The hollow, yet flexible, feathers consist of layers that are interlocked in an astonishing design of nature. The tips of the feathers at the ends of the wings are tapered which helps reduce turbulence as air currents pass over the end of the wings. All of these attributes combined ensure a smooth ride.

God gave a beautiful analogy about the kind of flight we can expect if we wait upon Him. There always will be turbulent times in life. There will be times when we feel we cannot make it. But, if we turn these times over to Him and wait for Him to accomplish His perfect will through them, we will enjoy a smooth ride. As my father-in-law would say, it is time for us to "hurry up and *wait!*"

Application:
1) In what areas of your life do you find the most difficulty waiting upon the Lord?
2) What is one thing you can do toward the goal of learning to wait upon the Lord?

PRAY and quiet yourself long enough to hear from God, even if it requires a little wait.

DEVOTIONAL FOR CHAPTER FIVE

Day Six

Scripture Reading: John 18:28-36; Hebrews 11:8-10

Verse of the Day: *Jesus replied, "Foxes have holes and birds of the air have nests, but the Son of Man has no place to lay his head"* (Matthew 8:20).

The verse of the day often has saddened my heart. In the past, I have wanted to cry whenever I thought of Jesus as a homeless person. But one day it occurred to me that there is a greater meaning to this verse.

I am sure that as an itinerant rabbi, Jesus must have felt as if He had no place to call home. He traveled many miles teaching about the truth of His Father's kingdom. We read of Him staying in the home of friends such as Mary, Martha, and Lazarus and returning to His family's home in Nazareth. However, there is no mention of His having a home of His own. Even the animals and fowl had their own homes, but not our Savior.

I came to the conclusion that the reason Jesus did not feel He had a place to call home was because He realized this world was not where He really belonged. It was His temporary address.

In that sense, we should be "homeless" people. We are placed in this world merely to prepare for the wonderful place that is really our home—heaven. As the old gospel song says, "This world is not my home. I'm only passing through."

According to Hebrews 11:8-10, Abraham realized this. He lived his life on earth looking forward to a city *whose architect and builder is God*. He could enjoy the beauty of this world, as well as endure its hardships, because he understood that he was "homeless" *here* while preparing for *there*. Very often homeless people came to our door for help.

This same realization is what allowed Jesus to stand before Pontius Pilate and proclaim in His very own words, *"My kingdom is not of this world"* (John 18:36).

Once we lived beside the church where my husband served as

pastor in the downtown section of our city. Very often homeless people came to our door for help. Truly, many of them had no place to lay their heads. As we offered physical help to them, we also shared how to have a relationship with God through Jesus Christ. Several responded by opening their hearts to the Savior.

It fills my heart with great joy to realize that though they are homeless, they are now also "homeless." Even though they have no place to lay their heads here, they one day will have a mansion as their real home!

Application:
1) Where do you belong? Have you established your new address in heaven?
2) If so, praise God and share the good news with as many others as you can.
3) If not, will you consider becoming a "homeless" person today?

PRAY and thank God for preparing a new home for all who receive Him.

DEVOTIONAL FOR CHAPTER FIVE

Day Seven

Scripture Reading: I Corinthians 15:35-58

Verse of the Day: *All flesh is not the same: Men have one kind of flesh, animals have another, birds another and fish another* (I Corinthians 15:39).

The church at Corinth raised some of the same questions we ponder today. How can the dead be resurrected? What kind of body will a resurrected person have? Paul's strong reply is that the Corinthians could find these answers by observing the nature around them. Their world was full of parallels to answer these questions, as is ours.

First, there are examples shown by seeds. A seed cannot

produce new life until it first dies. A seed is different from the new plant that springs forth with life. God is the One who gives each seed its own body and causes a plant to rise from the seed's death.

Next, there are examples shown by animals. Just as God gave each animal its own body (*flesh*), He surely is able to change a man's body from physical into spiritual.

Finally, there are examples shown by the heavenly bodies. God made the heavenly bodies different from earthly bodies, and different from each other. He gave each of them their own glory. God also will give each believer a resurrected body with its own glory.

Paul clearly shows that the principles of nature point to the mystery of the resurrection of man. From the seed we learn that our earthly bodies will die, and our spiritual bodies will be raised. From the differences among the animals, we learn that the composition of our resurrected bodies will be different from the composition of our earthly bodies. From the various glories among the heavenly bodies we learn that the glory of man's resurrected body will be different from the glory of man's earthly body.

Paul offers an explanation of the differences between our future resurrected bodies and our present earthly ones. Our resurrected bodies will be incorruptible and never will deteriorate. They will not be dishonorable, but glorious and full of perfect light. They will not be weak, but strong and powerful. Although they will retain those qualities which make us recognizable, they will somehow be changed into a different composition prepared for a different dimension—heaven.

Paul concludes by assuring that these changes will take place when Christ comes for all true believers at what has come to be known as "the rapture." There is urgency in Paul's writings for Christians to remain prepared for that glorious day.

Thank you, Paul, for answering those questions and giving such powerful insights concerning the resurrection to the church at Corinth and to us, two thousand years later.

Application:
1) Which example from nature means the most to you? Why?
2) What are you doing to remain spiritually prepared for that glorious day?

PRAY and thank God in advance for the resurrected body you will have one day.

CHAPTER SIX

BIBLICAL APPLICATION

The Sixth and Final Day of Creation

(Genesis 1:24-31)

24 And God said, "Let the land produce living creatures according to their kinds: livestock, creatures that move along the ground, and wild animals, each according to its kind." And it was so. 25 God made the wild animals according to their kinds, the livestock according to their kinds, and all creatures that move along the ground according to their kinds. And God saw that it was good.

26 Then God said, "Let us make man in our image, in our likeness, and let them rule over the fish of the sea and the birds of the air, over the livestock, over all the earth, and over all the creatures that move along the ground." 27 So God created man in his own image, in the image of God he created him; male and female he created them.

28 God blessed them and said to them, "Be fruitful and increase in number; fill the earth and subdue it. Rule over the fish of the sea and the birds of the air and all the creatures that move on the ground."

29 Then God said, "I give you every seed-bearing plant on the face of the whole earth and every tree that has fruit with seed in it. They will be yours for food. 30 And to all the beasts of the earth and all the birds of the air and all the creatures that move on the ground—everything that has the breath of life in it—I give every

green plant for food." And it was so.
31 God saw all that he had made, and it was very good. And there was evening, and there was morning—the sixth day.

The final day of the world's creation had arrived. Each thing created up to this point reached its culmination on the sixth day. Like a carefully designed set awaiting the opening curtain and the appearance of the leading character, the world was prepared for God's ultimate act of creation.

On **day one**, light and happiness were summoned into being.
On the **second day**, the waters were separated into atmosphere and waters on earth.
On the **third day**, dry land appeared; three categories of vegetation were created.
On the **fourth day**, the sun, moon, and stars were placed in the heavens.
On the **fifth day**, the first living beings, fish and fowl, were placed in their abodes.

Everything was in its intended order. The pristine world was bathed in light and happiness. Pure air; crystal clean streams, rivers, lakes, and seas; lush vegetation; majestic designations of times and seasons in the heavens; teeming schools of fish swimming in the waters and flocks of fowl flying in unpolluted skies played their parts in making the world a perfect place. It was perfect, but not complete until this final day of creation.

The sixth day was characterized by a double creation, corresponding to the double creations of the third day—dry land and plant life. On the sixth day, three categories of animals and then, man, were created to dwell on the dry land and subsist on the plant life.

And God said, "Let the land produce living creatures according to their kinds" (Genesis 1:24a). The Hebrew words for *living creature* are *nephesh chayyah* meaning "animated (merry, running, multitude) beings." This verse ends with *livestock and creatures that move along the ground, and wild animals, each according to its kind.* This conclusion to Genesis 1:24 clearly subdivides the animated beings, or land animals, into three well-defined categories.

I. LIVESTOCK (CATTLE)

Livestock (*cattle* in the King James Version) in Hebrew is *behemah* "the dumb, or mute, animal." Once again we are reminded that everything God does has a purpose. *Livestock* were the only "clean" land animals created, according to the description of clean land animals given in Deuteronomy 14:6. To be considered clean, an animal has to have split hooves and chew its cud. *Livestock* are the only animals that meet these criteria.

The significance of this rests in the fact that only clean animals could be used for sacrifice. Remember that Noah was instructed to take only one pair of unclean animals, but seven pairs of clean animals, onto the ark? Not only were the clean animals to be used for food after the flood, they were also the only ones appropriate for sacrifice.

In the creation of the *livestock*, and the later declaration that only they are considered clean, we have a beautiful foreshadowing of the coming Messiah. I often wondered why God created animals on the same day as man. It seemed to me that man would have been created on a separate day because of his uniqueness and the fact that he was given dominion over all other creations. In fact, scripture informs us that God made man *a little lower than the heavenly beings* (Psalm 8:5), or *angels* (Hebrews 2:7).

Then it occurred to me that God, the Master of thematic instruction, had once again employed foreshadowing on this final day of creation. He first summoned *livestock*, the only clean land animals suitable for sacrifice, from the dry land. Sheep are a part of this class because they have split hooves and chew their cuds. Throughout scripture, sheep, rams, and lambs were considered special animals for sacrifice.

This final day of creation was a beautiful example of foreshadowing when the lamb and man were created on the same day. God knew that one day He would be offered as the ultimate sacrifice. Jesus, who is both the Lamb of God and the Son of Man, would die once and for all as the eternal sacrifice for sin. Even the fact that the word "sheep" is both singular and plural points to the fact that a Sheep would be the ultimate sacrifice for His sheep.

As previously mentioned the Hebrew word for *livestock (cattle)* means "a dumb (mute) animal." Since sheep are in the cattle family, they are also known as "dumb, or mute, animals." Isaiah 53:7 records the following prophecy concerning the Messiah, *"He was oppressed and afflicted, yet he did not open his mouth; he was led like a lamb to the slaughter, and as a sheep before her shearers is silent [dumb in the King James Version], so he did not open his mouth."*

The night Jesus was falsely accused and unfairly tried is described in the Gospels. In Mark 15:3-5 it is recorded, *"The chief priests accused him of many things. So again Pilate asked him, 'Aren't you going to answer? See how many things they are accusing you of.' But Jesus still made no reply, and Pilate was amazed."* Truly He was the mute sacrificial Lamb who was brought as a sheep to the slaughter!

The Passover Lamb

Another poignant picture painted by foreshadowing can be found in the requirements of the Passover lamb as described in Exodus 12 and Deuteronomy 16. The life and death of Jesus of Nazareth—God in the flesh—explicitly fulfill each requirement. The requirements of the Passover lamb from the Torah, and the fulfillment by Jesus as recorded in the New Testament are as follows:

Requirement of the Passover Lamb
1. The lamb was to be without spot or blemish (Exodus 12:5).
Fulfillment in Jesus
1. Jesus was declared to be without fault, blemish or spot.
   Pilate. . . said, "I find no basis for a charge against him" (John 18:38).
   For you know that it was not with perishable things such as silver or gold that you were redeemed from the empty way of life handed down to you from your forefathers, but with the precious blood of Christ, a lamb without blemish or defect (I Peter 1:18,19).

Requirement of the Passover Lamb
2. The lamb was to be a male, and a lamb of the first year (Exodus 12:5).

Fulfillment in Jesus
2. Jesus was a male, and was the firstborn.

. . . and she gave birth to her firstborn, a son. She wrapped him in cloths, and placed him in a manger, because there was no room for them in the inn (Luke 2:7).

Requirement of the Passover Lamb
3. The lamb was to be brought into the house for four days (Exodus 12:3,6).

Fulfillment in Jesus
3. Jesus was in Jerusalem prior to His death, ministering in the house of God, for four days.

The crowds that went ahead of him and those that followed, shouted, " Hosanna to the Son of David!" "Blessed is he who comes in the name of the Lord!" "Hosanna in the highest!" (Matthew 21:9)

The blind and the lame came to him at the temple, and he healed them (Matthew 21:14).

Requirement of the Passover Lamb
4. The lamb was to be killed in the evening, by all the people of the community (Exodus 12:6).

Fulfillment in Jesus
4. Jesus died on the cross at 3:00 p.m., the time of the evening sacrifice.

About the ninth hour Jesus cried out in a loud voice, ". . . My God, my God, why have you forsaken me?" (Matthew 27:45)

And when Jesus had cried out again in a loud voice, he gave up his spirit (Matthew 27:50).

All the people of the community killed Jesus.

The kings of the earth take their stand and the rulers gather together against the Lord and against his Anointed One. Indeed Herod and Pontius Pilate met together with the Gentiles and the people of Israel in this city to conspire against your holy servant Jesus, whom you anointed (Acts 4:26,27).

Requirement of the Passover Lamb

5. The blood of the lamb was to be applied to the doorposts of the house (Exodus 12:7).

Fulfillment in Jesus

5. Jesus is the door. His blood allows us access into the household of God.

I am the door: by me if any man enter in, he shall be saved. . . (John 10:9 KJV).

For through him we both have access to the Father by one Spirit. Consequently, you are no longer foreigners and aliens, but fellow citizens with God's people and members of God's household. . . (Ephesians 2:18,19).

Requirement of the Passover Lamb

6. The lamb was to be roasted with fire and eaten in the same night (Exodus 12:8).

According to the Mishnah, the lamb was roasted on an upright pomegranate stick.

Fulfillment in Jesus

6. Throughout the Bible, fire is associated with judgment. The Gospels record that Jesus was arrested, tried, judged, and killed on an upright stake (a tree) within one night. (The biblical day goes from sundown to sundown, or approximately 6:00 p.m. one day to 6:00 p.m. the next day.)

The body and the blood of the lamb are associated with the body and blood of Jesus.

While they were eating, Jesus took bread, gave thanks and broke it, and gave it to his disciples, saying, "Take and eat; this is my body" (Matthew 26:26).

Then he took the cup, gave thanks and offered it to them saying, "Drink from it, all of you. This is my blood of the covenant, which is poured out for many for the forgiveness of sins" (Matthew 26:27,28).

Requirement of the Passover Lamb

7. The lamb had to be eaten in haste, with loins girded, shoes on, and staff in hand (Exodus 12:11).

Fulfillment in Jesus

7. Many passages throughout the gospels confirm that Jesus was arrested, tried, and killed hastily (Matthew 26:1-28:20; Mark 14:1-16:20; Luke 22:1-24:53; John 13:1-21:25).

Requirement of the Passover Lamb

8. The Passover lamb was to be eaten only by those who were circumcised (Exodus 12:43-48).

Fulfillment in Jesus

8. Through Jesus, our Passover Lamb, the Spirit of God circumcises our hearts.

   A man is not a Jew if he is only one outwardly, nor is circumcision merely outward and physical. No, a man is a Jew if he is one inwardly; and circumcision is circumcision of the heart, by the Spirit, not by the written code. . . (Romans 2:28,29).

Requirement of the Passover Lamb

9. The Passover lamb was to have no broken bones (Exodus 12:46).

Fulfillment in Jesus

9. When Jesus was crucified, the Roman soldiers broke the legs of the two thieves on either side of Him, but they did not break His bones.

   But when they came to Jesus and found that he was already dead, they did not break his legs (John 19:33).

Requirement of the Passover Lamb

10. In addition to the requirements for the original Passover, God gave instructions for future Passover observances. The lamb was to be killed in the place where God would choose to place His name (Deuteronomy 16:2,6). According to II Kings 21:4, God placed His name in Jerusalem. Even the typography of Jerusalem forms the Hebrew letter *shin* (ש), which in Hebrew thought represents *Shaddai*, "Almighty God."

Fulfillment in Jesus

10. Jesus was crucified in Jerusalem.

   After Jesus had said this, he went on ahead, going up to

Jerusalem (Luke 19:28).
And so Jesus also suffered outside the city [Jerusalem] *gate to make the people holy through his own blood* (Hebrews 13:12).

According to Jewish writings and traditions, at the third hour (9:00 a.m.) on Passover day the high priest ascended the altar and tied the Passover lamb representing the nation of Israel on the altar so all could see. We are told of Jesus in Mark 15:25, *It was the third hour when they crucified him.* Jesus' crucifixion also occurred on Passover day.

At the ninth hour (3:00 p.m.), the time of the evening sacrifice, the high priest once again ascended the altar, cut the throat of the lamb according to kosher slaughter, and said, "It is finished." In Matthew 27:46,50 we read that *about the ninth hour* [3:00 p.m.] *Jesus cried out in a loud voice, ". . . My God, my God, why have you forsaken Me?" And when Jesus had cried out again in a loud voice, he gave up his spirit.*

Also, in John 19:30, that final loud cry is recorded: *When he had received the drink, Jesus said, "It is finished." With that, he bowed his head and gave up his spirit.*

Yes, Jesus of Nazareth fulfilled every requirement of the Passover Lamb. Therefore, He could confidently say in Matthew 5:17, *"Do not think that I have come to abolish the Law or the Prophets; I have not come to abolish them but to fulfill them."*

Another beautiful foreshadowing verifies the fulfillment of the Law through Jesus, the Lamb of God. It originally was written on the hides of sacrificed lambs.

In addition to fulfilling the requirements of the Passover lamb, Jesus of Nazareth also fulfilled other requirements of every Jewish sacrificial offering. Isn't that amazing?

II. ANIMALS THAT MOVE ALONG THE GROUND (CREEPING THING)

The King James Version refers to *animals that move along the ground* as *creeping thing.* The Hebrew word for *creeping thing* is *remes* meaning "reptile or any other rapidly moving animal." It comes from *ramas*, which means "to glide swiftly, for example, to crawl or move with short steps." Therefore, a *creeping thing* is what its name implies, an animal that moves either without feet, or with feet that are hard to distinguish.

III. WILD ANIMALS (BEAST OF THE EARTH)

Wild animals are called *beast of the earth* in the King James Version. *Beast* in Hebrew is *chay*, meaning "alive; raw flesh; fresh; strong (wild)." These animals are carnivorous predators.

God summoned all three categories of land animals from the earth itself with the words ". . . *Let the land produce*. . . "(Genesis 1:24). Like fish and fowl, they were created in distinct order and species types. However, they were created from the earth or land and not from the previously existing animals.

Livestock, Animals that Move Along the Ground, Wild Animals

The Creator surveyed the work He had done thus far on the sixth day, and He was pleased. *And God saw that it was good* (Genesis 1:25b).

IV. MAN—THE CROWNING WORK OF CREATION

Yes, it was good! Everything was prepared carefully for the most dramatic moment of the week of creation, the advent of man. I remember how my husband and I planned for the birth of our daughters. The time of pregnancy had been a time of preparation. In addition to praying constantly for our baby, we designed and decorated the nursery. We bought the necessary baby items, and we chose a meaningful name. It seemed that during the time of expectation and preparation, every thought and action were in joyful anticipation of the birth of our baby.

I can only imagine the excitement God must have felt when He came to this point in the sixth day. His every thought and every action had been in joyful anticipation of this moment.

The importance of this event is indicated by the way that this act of creation is introduced. *Then God said, "Let us make man in our image, in our likeness. . . "* (Genesis 1:26a). In this verse we see that a heavenly council was held among the three persons of the Godhead—Father, Son, and Holy Spirit. There are those who feel that *us* in this verse refers to angels. Others feel that it refers to the newly created animals. However, neither angels nor animals can create out of nothingness. Only God can.

The reason for the heavenly consortium was the creation of man. He, Adam, was to be made in the *image* and *likeness* of God Himself. Exactly what that means has been an enigma throughout time. I have asked many ministerial friends to explain what they think it means to be made in the image of God. In response, I have been given many different replies.

Everything in the Bible is multi-dimensional, so I am sure there are many answers. Yet the discoveries I found to be most meaningful are in the words *image* and *likeness*. In Hebrew, *image* is *tselem* and it means "to shade (a shadow); a phantom, such as an illusion or resemblance." Thus, an image is a representative figure. *Likeness* in Hebrew is *demuwth*, which comes from *damah*, and means "resemblance; similitude."

We are made in the *image* and *likeness* of God—spirit, soul and body. The persons of the Godhead are One, yet each has distinctive characteristics. One does not exist without the other. God the Father, God the Son, and God the Holy Spirit exist as a unit.

The same is true of us as individuals. The spirit (spiritual), soul (mental and emotional), and body (physical) are one, yet each has distinctive characteristics. One does not exist without the other. The spirit, soul, and body exist as a unit.

The body (physical) is in the *image* of Jesus, who was the bodily form of God on earth: *The Word became flesh and made his dwelling among us* (John 1:14). *And being found in appearance as a man, He humbled Himself and became obedient to death—even death on a cross!* (Philippians 2:8)

The soul (mental and emotional) is in the *likeness* of God the Father. God's heart is filled with various emotions toward His creations, especially love: *Dear friends, let us love one another, for love comes from God* (I John 4:7). However, we also are told in scripture that there are times when He experiences anger: *The wrath of God is being revealed from heaven against all the godlessness and wickedness of men who suppress the truth by their wicked-*

ness (Romans 1:18), and even jealousy: . . . *for I, the Lord your God, am a jealous God*. . . (Exodus 20:5).

The spirit (spiritual) is in the *likeness* of God, the Holy Spirit. His characteristics are available also to those who have received His indwelling: *But the fruit of the Spirit is love, joy, peace, patience, kindness, goodness, faithfulness, gentleness, and self-control*. . . (Galatians 5:22-23). He is the One who convicts of sin: *When he comes, he will convict the world of guilt in regard to sin and righteousness and judgment* (John 16:8).

The Holy Spirit points the way of truth to the Father through the Son: *Jesus said, "But when he, the Spirit of truth, comes he will guide you into all truth*. . . *He will bring glory to me by taking from what is mine and making it known to you"* (John 16:13,14).

The Holy Spirit also spiritually intercedes on our behalves: *In the same way, the Spirit helps us in our weakness. We do not know what we ought to pray for, but the Spirit himself intercedes for us with groans that words cannot express* (Romans 8:26).

Being made in the *image* and *likeness* of God indicates an external as well as an internal dimension. What an awesome privilege to bear the *image* and *likeness* of God the Father, God the Son, and God the Holy Spirit!

Adam, the First Man

So God created man in His own image, in the image of God created He him. . . (Genesis 1:27). Once again the Hebrew word *bara* is used for *created*, indicating that a brand new creation was formed. We have seen this word used twice before—first, when God created the heaven and earth and next, when the first living beings (fish and fowl) were created. Finally, it is used when the ultimate act of creation—man—is placed in the world.

God carefully fashioned man in His own image. A beautiful picture of how this was done is painted in Genesis 2:7, . . . *the Lord God formed the man from the dust of the ground and breathed into his nostrils the breath of life, and the man became a living being*. God took the dust of the ground and constructed the first man. This truth is confirmed through research showing that the basic elements that comprise man are the same as those found in the earth.

God then breathed into his nostrils. The Hebrew word used here for *breathed* is *naphach,* which literally means "to blow hard; to inflate."

That which was blown into man's nostrils separated him from the previous creations. It was the *breath of life, neshamah,* "vital breath, and divine inspiration; spirit." Animals had been given mental and emotional capabilities, but only man was given a spirit. He alone can commune with God in the spiritual sense.

God called the first man *Adam.* Although it is not mentioned specifically when God named him, the first reference to his name is found in Genesis 2:19 when God brought the animals before Adam to receive their various names.

Scholars have debated for years the intended meaning of Adam's name. Some explanations, using various etymologies, are that his name refers to his color; his shiny appearance; his origin from the earth; his compactness; or his resemblance to God.

The Hebrew word *Adam* means—"ruddy (red); a human being; mankind." It comes from the word that means "to show blood in the face, for example, to be flush or turn rosy; to be dyed or made red; ruddy."

I believe that once again God employed foreshadowing even in the name He gave the first man, indicating that one day He would come to earth in the form of a man, and would "show blood in the face." He would be "made red" as His blood atoned for all of mankind. God, the Son, would be made red, so that our sins could be made white: *"Come now, let us reason together," says the Lord. "Though your sins are like scarlet, they shall be as white as snow; though they are red as crimson, they shall be like wool"* (Isaiah 1:18).

The Perfection of the First Man

Probably we have all wondered what Adam, the first human being created, was like. Since he was created without sin and because no generational imperfections had been passed down to him, he was the epitome of what God intended for us all to be. He was perfect in spirit, soul, and body.

Body (Physical)

Adam's physical make-up was perfect. All of his senses were developed to the fullest degree. Scientists say that we see only about 5% of the total color scheme in the world, but Adam was able to see every beautiful, dazzling color in God's perfect world!

We are told that today we hear only about 2% of the sound patterns in the world. Researchers now are aware of the fact that every living cell emits a type of music all its own. Adam was able to hear the harmonious sounds of a world filled with living beings.

The 100+ trillion cells in Adam's body were perfect. He did not experience sickness, pain, or weakness. He was strong, agile, and beautiful to behold.

Adam probably shone with brilliance and light that is hidden from us today. Modern research has proven that pure raw foods cause the forward and reverse spin of the electrons in the cells to travel in a straight line, producing light. Since Adam's diet consisted of these pure, light-producing foods, he probably radiated an unadulterated internal light.

In addition, because of his relationship with God, he reflected the brilliance of God! Moses had to cover his face after he met with God on the mountain because he shone so brightly the people could not bear to look directly at him (Exodus 34:29-35). How much more this would have been true of Adam before sin entered his life and separated him from the light of God's glory!

Soul (Mental and Emotional)

It has been estimated that today mankind uses less than 10% of the potential ability of the brain. (Some researchers feel it is only around 1%.) Adam used his brain's full potential. We cannot imagine how intelligent he was.

We are told in Genesis 2:19 that God brought the animals to Adam . . . *to see what he would name them; and whatever the man called each living creature, that was its name*. It has been estimated that today, there are more than 3,500 different mammals, 5,500 reptiles and amphibians, and over 8,600 birds in existence, and possibly there were even more in Adam's day. Yet, he was so intelligent and had such a vast vocabulary, he was able to assign each of them a name.

Apparently Adam (and Eve) had the ability of communicating with the animals. In Genesis 3:1-6, Eve somehow had a dialogue with the serpent.

Not only was Adam extraordinarily intelligent, prior to sinning, his emotions were in a perfected state. He knew no sorrow, depression, guilt, fear nor shame. He did not experience these emotions until after he fell from his sinless condition.

Spirit (Spiritual)

Adam was created without sin, so he was able to commune intimately with God. He heard God's voice and commandments clearly, and therefore understood God's perfect will for his life: *And the Lord God commanded the man, "You are free to eat from any tree in the garden; but you must not eat from the tree of the knowledge of good and evil, for when you eat of it you will surely die"* (Genesis 2:16,17).

Repeatedly God deemed His creations *good*. The narrative of each day's creative activities, with the exception of the second day, ends with phrases such as *and God saw that it was good*. Therefore, Adam knew only that which was good. He experienced physical life and the fruit of the Spirit—*love, joy, peace, patience, kindness, goodness, faithfulness, gentleness, and self-control*—in abundant measure.

Since God is good, it is His heart's desire that all people know His goodness. God expressed this desire when He told Adam that he could eat freely of every tree in the garden except *from the tree of the knowledge of good and evil* (Genesis 2:17). God understood the pain that the experience of evil would cause. As soon as Adam and Eve chose to eat of the tree of the knowledge of good and evil, the presence of evil became a part of them and each subsequent generation thereafter.

Sin separates us from intimacy with God: *If I had cherished sin in my heart, the Lord would not have listened* (Psalm 66:18). Prior to making the choice that allowed iniquity into his heart, Adam walked and talked with God, and heard directly from Him.

God gave Adam the freedom to choose between good and evil. The Creator clearly displayed Himself through all that was good, and forbade only what would hide His goodness. Adam was not a mere puppet. He was a spiritual being capable of making choices that would reward him with the awareness of God's presence, or punish him with separation from the awareness of God's presence. Adam had the choice of living in the goodness of God's light, or choosing evil by turning from God's light.

From the moment Adam sinned, he knew the anguish of his new knowledge of evil. Along with this knowledge came the negative thoughts and emotions from which he had been protected. Lust, pride, deceit, and impurity were now a part of him. The resulting feelings of fear, shame, and guilt accompanied them.

We should be very mindful of the fact that if Adam, who originally lived in a perfect relationship with God, chose to know evil, we today must be even more careful. We, unlike Adam, are born in a sinful state. We can be aware of God's presence only as we seek Him through obedience to the light of His Word: *Live as children of light (for the fruit of the light consists in all goodness, righteousness and truth) and find out what pleases the Lord* (Ephesians 5:8-10). Through obeying Him we will find His goodness, which is His perfect will for our lives.

The Creation of Woman

. . . male and female he created them (Genesis 1:27). The Creation narrative recorded in the first chapter of Genesis does not supply the details of the creation of Eve, the first woman. However, a beautifully descriptive narrative is given in Genesis 2:20-25 as follows:

> *So the man gave names to all the livestock, the birds of the air and all the beasts of the field. But for Adam no suitable helper was found. So the Lord God caused the man to fall into a deep sleep: and while he was sleeping, he took one of the man's ribs and closed up the place with flesh. Then the Lord God made a woman from the rib he had taken out of the man, and he brought her to the man. The man said, "This is now bone of my bones and flesh of my flesh; she shall be called 'woman,' for she was taken out of man." For this reason a man will leave his father and mother and be united to his wife, and they will become one flesh. The man and his wife were both naked, and they felt no shame.*

Thus unfolds the story of the first wedding. God's primary institution, the family, was formed in this union.

The animals Adam named had mates, but he was the only one of his kind. He had no one who could compare to him or relate to him as a person.

God lovingly brought Eve into existence from Adam. The sleep that Adam fell into was much more than normal sleep. It is the Hebrew word *tardemah,* "to be languid (without energy; weak); to remain long in sleep" and it figuratively refers to death. Adam fell into a long, deep, unconscious sleep. The Hebrew word for *rib* is *tsela* meaning, in this case, "rib (as curved); side (of a person)."

The following has been noted beautifully:

> *God did not take Eve from Adam's feet, that she might be trampled by him; nor did God take Eve from Adam's head, that she might be mastered by him; but God took Eve from Adam's side, under his arm, that she might be protected by him; and close to his heart, that she might be loved by him.*

The Hebrew word for *Eve* is *Chavvah,* which not only means "the first woman," but also "life-giver." As Adam's helper, she would be also the life-giver of the children who would precede all generations to come.

The Divine Commission

God blessed them and said to them, "Be fruitful and increase in number; fill the earth and subdue it. Rule over the fish of the sea and the birds of the air and over every living creature that moves on the ground" (Genesis 1:28).

God gave Adam and Eve dominion over the animals in the exact order in which they had been created—fish, fowl, and land animals. The first human couple also was given dominion over all the earth, which essentially means that Adam and Eve were given reign or rule over the earth and its inhabitants. The other creations were to be in subjection to them.

They were expected to use their intelligence and their abilities to be good stewards of the wonderful world in which they lived. In addition, they were given the use of the vast resources in the world to meet their needs.

This place of honor above the other creations was yet another way in which God showed how precious mankind is to Him. In Psalm 8:4-9, David writes as follows:

> *...what is man that you are mindful of him, the son of man that you care for him? You made him a little lower than the heavenly beings and crowned him with glory and honor. You made him ruler over the works of your hands; you put everything under his feet: all flocks and herds, and the beasts of the field, the birds of the air, and the fish of the sea, all that swim the paths of the seas. O Lord, our Lord, how majestic is your name in all the earth!*

What a wonderful honor God bestowed upon Adam when he was placed in esteem second only to the angels! We are told in the book of Hebrews that when Jesus came to earth as a man, He who had been far superior to the angels took on a form that was lower than the angels: *But we see Jesus, who was made a little lower than the angels, now crowned with glory and honor because he suffered death, so that by the grace of God he might taste death for everyone* (Hebrews 2:9).

Jesus, God in the flesh, gave up the glories of heaven to come to earth to die for mankind. What greater honor could be given to us, the created, than for the Creator to die in place of each of us?

The Blessing

God blessed them and said to them, "Be fruitful and increase in number; fill the earth. . . " (Genesis 1:28). Again, as in the preceding chapter regarding fish and fowl, there is a special meaning in the Hebrew word for *blessed, barak*, which means "to kneel down (as an act of adoration); praise; salute; thank." God's blessing of Adam and Eve was a holy moment in time.

Many Jewish rabbis teach that this blessing was a twofold act. First, the actual blessing of Adam and Eve took place. Some scholars feel this was a part of their marriage ceremony.

Secondly, a special blessing for the proliferation of their species was pronounced upon them. They were to be fruitful and multiply so they could replenish the earth. The first man and woman were not created in schools, flocks, or herds as the other animals. They were created as divinely sculpted individuals.

Sages say that the pronouncement to be fruitful and multiply was not only a blessing, but also the first of the 613 commandments in the Torah. It was a positive command, which carried with it special blessings.

The Provision

The ideal man and the ideal woman were placed in an ideal environment. With every resource at their command, God further disclosed His perfect will for their lives.

> *Then God said, "I give you every seed-bearing plant on the face of the whole earth and every tree that has fruit with seed in it. They will be yours for food. And to all the beasts of the earth and all the birds of the air and all the creatures that move on the ground— everything that has the breath of life in it—I give every green plant for food." And it was so* (Genesis 1:29,30).

The Creator lovingly explained to Adam and Eve that all the vegetables and fruits He had created were provided for their food. God also explained that He had provided the green vegetation for the animals. The ideal man and the ideal woman had been placed in the ideal environment with the ideal diet. What could be more wonderful?

The Benediction

God saw all that he had made, and it was very good (Genesis 1:31). Once again the Creator surveyed His world. This time, He not only surveyed the creations of the sixth day, but also the creations of the previous five days. Each was good individually, and all were good collectively. His work was now complete.

In an orderly and precise way, He had called forth resources, living beings, and mankind. The omnipotent, omniscient, omnipresent God created the world, then filled it sequentially with things that were necessary to sustain life.

As He looked upon the completed work of creation, the scripture says that God was pleased. Each creation previously had been deemed *good*. Now all of creation was deemed more than *good*. It was *very good. And there was evening, and there was morning—the sixth day* (Genesis 1:31).

NUTRITIONAL APPLICATION

Clean and Unclean Animals

As was presented in Chapter Five, the understanding of clean and unclean animals had been in place long before the nation of Israel was established. Noah, a Gentile, was instructed by God to take seven pairs of clean animals and one pair of unclean animals on the ark. After the flood, when the eating of meat became permissible, Noah and his family had enough clean animals to present for sacrifice and to replenish their species on earth. It is possible that their meat consumption consisted of animals that had been sacrificed and burned on the altar since God later permitted the priests to do so.

Later, the nation of Israel was established through Abraham. Then, during the time of Moses, God gave the Law, or Torah, to the Israelites at Mt. Sinai. The instructions contained in the Torah give a written account of which animals were considered clean and unclean.

Only clean animals could be eaten. According to Deuteronomy 14:3-8; 19,20 the following is taught:

> *Do not eat any detestable thing. These are the animals you may eat: the ox, the sheep, the goat, the deer, the gazelle, the roe deer, the wild goat, the ibex* [wild mountain goat], *and antelope and the mountain sheep. You may eat any animal that has a split hoof divided in two and that chews the cud. However, of those that chew the cud or that have a split hoof completely divided you may not eat the camel, the*

rabbit or the coney [a small, rodent-like animal with hooves.]. *Although they chew the cud, they do not have a split hoof; they are ceremonially unclean for you. The pig is also unclean; although it has a split hoof, it does not chew the cud. You are not to eat their meat or touch their carcasses...All flying insects that swarm are unclean to you; do not eat them. But any winged creature that is clean you may eat.*

Camels, rabbits, coneys, and pigs were excluded from the clean list for a purpose; they did not meet both criteria. Even though camels, rabbits, and coneys chew their cuds, they do not have split hooves. On the other hand, pigs have split hooves, but do not chew their cuds. To qualify as clean, an animal had to possess both qualities.

In looking at the list of clean animals—ox, sheep, goat, deer, gazelle, ibex, antelope—we see that they all are considered a part of the livestock (cattle) family. The first animals created from the land on the sixth day are the only animals that were both suitable for religious ceremony and for dietary purposes.

Toxicity of Unclean Animals

A landmark study was conducted at Johns Hopkins University in 1953 which confirmed the validity of the instructions God had given in the Torah thousands of years earlier. Dr. David Macht studied the toxic effects of animal flesh on a controlled growth culture. Toxic flesh slowed the growth rate of the culture. Everything that tested below the growth rate of 75% was considered toxic.

Amazingly, all the clean animals from the Bible were shown to have averages well above 75%. That included fish with fins and scales, birds not from the forbidden list, land animals that chewed their cuds and had split hooves (calf, ox, deer, goat, and sheep), and winged insects that hopped with four legs (as opposed to those that swarm).

Every single animal that was tested on God's list of unclean animals had an average below 75%. The animals God told us to avoid in our diets have toxic flesh!

Another amazing fact was confirmed through Dr. Macht's

research project. As was presented earlier, when the eating of meat became permissible, God made sure that Noah and his family understood they were not to eat the blood of animals: *But you must not eat meat that has its lifeblood still in it* (Genesis 9:4).

The Creation Diet repeatedly has reiterated the fact from Leviticus 17:14 that *the life of every creature is in its blood*. The blood transports both life-giving nutrients to the cells, and carries toxins away from the cells for removal as waste. Therefore, without blood, there is no life.

Dr. Macht found in his study of animal toxicity that the blood of animals is even more toxic than their flesh. God knew this, so when He gave permission to eat meat, He clearly stated that no blood from the animals was to be eaten.

There are several interesting facts concerning the livestock or cattle class of clean animals. In their natural states, animals in the cattle class are herbivorous or granivorous, eating only vegetation. Secondly, none of them is considered a predator (an animal that preys on other animals). When they are allowed to graze they do not carry the diseases in their bodies that predators, which consume the bloody flesh of other animals, do.

Creatures that move along the ground and *wild animals* are either carnivorous (meat eating) or omnivorous (both meat and plant eating). They do not meet the two criteria of having split hooves and chewing the cud. Therefore, they are unclean both for religious and dietary purposes.

I. LIVESTOCK (CATTLE)

It is important to note that in biblical days, meats from this category were "special occasion" entrees for most people. The average person did not consume them on a daily basis. The following examples illustrate that fact:

- Roasted lamb was served during Passover and at other religious feasts.
- Jesus told through a parable that when the prodigal son returned home, the father instructed the servant, *"Bring the fatted calf, and kill it. Let's have a feast and celebrate"*

(Luke 15:23). This demonstrates that beef was reserved for a time of rejoicing.

- Meat from this category was used to show hospitality. When Abraham was visited by heavenly guests we are told that Abraham *ran to the herd and selected a choice, tender calf and gave it to a servant who hurried to prepare it"* (Genesis 18:7).

- Meat from the cattle category was considered to be such a delicacy, Isaac asked Esau to prepare some for what he thought was a dying wish: *Now then, get your weapons— your quiver and bow—and go out to the open country to hunt some wild game [venison KJV] for me. Prepare me the kind of tasty food I like and bring it to me to eat, so that I may give you my blessing before I die* (Genesis 27:3,4).

Since beef is the most consumed meat from the livestock class in America, the nutritional application in this chapter of The Creation Diet will center on cattle. In its unadulterated state, beef contains protein, iron, zinc and various vitamins.

It also contains some Omega 3 fatty acids. As was presented in Chapter Five, Omega 3 fatty acids produce numerous beneficial functions in the body.

When cattle are allowed to graze naturally, they ingest grasses and grains that are healthful. The unique design of their digestive system is especially interesting.

The stomach of a cow contains four rumination pouches. Inside each pouch are various kinds of friendly bacteria that help to digest the grasses and grains. As these bacteria compete for the nutrients that are introduced into each pouch, they crowd out the harmful elements and help to destroy toxins before they reach the flesh of the cow.

CHOICES THAT DIMINISH THE BENEFITS OF CATTLE

In today's world of big business, we have strayed far from God's original design. There are numerous health risks associated with how cows are raised, slaughtered, and processed. In general, sheep are allowed to roam and graze rather than being raised on factory farms. However, in most instances, this is not the case with cows.

Adulteration of Livestock Food Sources

Cows are generally docile animals which graze on grass and other vegetation. However, during this day of factory farmed livestock, cows are transported to feedlots which might house thousands of cows. They are confined to small concrete stalls with slatted metal floors, where they are so crowded they do not have room to move.

Their natural instinct to graze is suppressed as they are given a steady diet of livestock food. This "food" contains such things as poultry litter, artificial hay, shredded scraps of paper, sawdust, tallow, and grease. The purpose of the cattle feed is to fatten the animals quickly for market.

Mad Cow Disease

Bovine Spongiform Encephalopathy, also known as Mad Cow Disease, is a fatal neurological disease. It is believed to have been transmitted by livestock feed containing slaughtered parts from sheep and cows, including infected brain tissue.

The most common form of Mad Cow Disease is Creutzfeidt-Jakob Disease, a form that can be transmitted to humans who eat the meat of infected cows. The infectious agent is a protein fragment unlike any other known germ, and it is remarkably strong and hard to destroy. In fact, there is no cure for Mad Cow Disease at the present, and the incubation period from exposure to symptoms can be as long as 10-15 years.

It is a major violation of the law of nature to feed cattle meat to other cattle. For some time the carcasses of dead cows were mixed with carcasses of other animals and added to livestock feed. We then began reaping the grim results of violating God's design. The split-hoofed, cud-chewing, "clean" animals from the cattle category are vegetarian animals by nature. We as humans simply cannot improve on God's natural creations.

In this case, thankfully, in 1997 the Food and Drug Administration put into effect a ban on the use of ruminant (cattle) animal feed containing any parts of other ruminant animals.

Chemical Additives and Injections

As with the poultry industry discussed in Chapter Five, the cattle industry has a goal to get the animals and their products to market as quickly and cheaply as possible. One of their aims is to fatten the animals that will be slaughtered for meat since weight determines the market price. Another intent is to keep milk cows producing as much milk as possible for dairy products.

Unfortunately, in order to accomplish their goals the cattle are exposed to a constant barrage of toxic chemicals that enter their systems. Many of these toxins are stored in their flesh, and passed on to those who eat the animals and/or their products.

Young cattle are shipped primarily by truck to feed lots where they spend the remainder of their lives. The transport to these feed lots can be devastating to the young cows. Often they go without food and water for several days in crowded conditions as they are being moved. Ventilation is poor and often temperatures are severe. There is a high risk of death due to a form of pneumonia appropriately called "shipping fever." To prevent loss of animals, livestock producers use antibiotics to treat shipping fever.

In his book, <u>Diet for a New America</u>, John Robbins reveals the dangers of chloramphenicol, the most common antibiotic used to treat shipping fever. He points out that it can be highly dangerous to humans. Even a small amount can cause disease and/or death in human beings who are susceptible to it.

When the young cows arrive at the feed lots they are dipped in a trough of insecticides to kill parasites that thrive on factory farms. They are injected with various chemicals, including growth stimulants and hormones to fatten them quickly. These growth hormones, which were first introduced into livestock production after World War II, are passed to humans through meat and dairy products.

As a result, we find a generation of people who are experiencing hormonal imbalances and a myriad of sexual behavior disorders. In fact, the age of menses of American girls has dropped from around 14 years of age a little over a generation ago to 8 to 9 years of age today. Everything from sexual deviancy to severe symptoms associated with premenstrual syndrome and menopause is increasing at alarming rates. Many of these conditions can be traced back to the combination of growth hormones passed onto humans from cattle meat plus what was already present in the human body.

Due to the fact that the cows are crowded into stalls and are not allowed to roam, their living conditions draw swarms of flies and other insects. So, livestock farmers add poisons, designed to kill insect larvae, to the cattle feed. After the cows eat the larvicides, they are passed through the digestive systems and excreted as poisonous manure to prevent insect breeding. The problem is that not all the chemicals pass through, and residues of toxins remain in the meat and by-products of the cattle.

When compounded with the toxins that are added to the cattle feed, humans are ingesting poisons at alarming rates. In fact, recent studies indicate that approximately 95% to 99% of toxic chemical residues in the American diet come from meat and dairy products.

Poor Choices When Shopping

When we eat meat from the cattle category, several things should be taken into consideration. First, choose lean cuts of meat. Factory farmed animals have a higher concentration of fat than pasture raised cattle. One reason is that they are confined to narrow stalls on the feed lots and are not able to move and exercise. Also, the additives in their feed as well as injections of growth hormones fatten them quickly.

The fat found in factory farmed animals is much more saturated than in pasture raised cows. One study revealed as much as 30 times more saturated fat. In addition, bulls are castrated (testicles removed) to produce steers, and steers have more saturated fat than bulls. Meats are graded according to fat content. Since steers have fat marbled through the flesh where it cannot be trimmed off, they bring a higher price. It is best to choose cuts that can be trimmed and not ones with fat marbled through the flesh.

When shopping, it is important to find sources where cattle are the following:

- Pasture raised
- Free from the use of chemicals (insecticides, antibiotics, growth stimulants, hormones, and pesticides)
- Fed organically grown food.

Many health food stores and some large grocery stores either carry these kinds of meats or will order them for you. Also, co-ops were discussed in Chapter Five. With a minimal number of participants (usually around fifteen), you can place bulk orders directly from farms or processors, then divide and distribute the meat among the members.

Methods of Cooking

As with all protein from animal sources, beef should be cooked on moderate to low heat. If grilling, keep at least six inches away from the source of heat.

MILK

The benefits of milk have been in question for some time. There are those who say neither milk nor dairy products made from milk should be consumed. Others laud that these products are full of protein, calcium and bone-building elements. Today's consumer is baffled by these conflicting messages.

It is true that there are many positive biblical references to milk. One example is that the Promised Land is referred to as *a land flowing with milk and honey* (Exodus 3:8). We read in Isaiah 55:1, *"Come all you who are thirsty, come to the waters; and you who have no money, come, buy and eat! Come, buy wine and milk without money and without cost."*

However, most of the milk consumed in biblical times came from goats rather than from cows. In Deuteronomy 32:14, God provided Jacob the following: *curds and milk from herd and flock and with fattened lambs and goats.*

In Proverbs 27:27 it is written, *"You will have plenty of goats' milk to feed you and your family and to nourish your servant girls."* Even Virgil wrote during the first century A.D., "Camel's, goat's, and ewe's milk is for humans, cow's milk for calves."

The protein molecules in cow's milk are much larger than in goat's milk. Consider the fact that the milk from a mother cow turns a small calf into a four hundred pound animal in a short time.

Out of the Mouths of Babes

The Bible indicates that during biblical times, infants drank milk and adults ate curds. In his writings, Paul repeatedly stated that milk was for babies and solid food was for adults. Humans are the only beings who continue to drink milk after they have been weaned. Also, we are the only ones who drink milk from another animal species. Animals in the natural only drink milk from their own species.

A human mother's milk is perfect in every way for a baby. It contains the proper balance of organic vitamins, minerals, carbohydrates, essential amino acids, and essential fatty acids. It also contains the perfect concentration of calories, amino acids and enzymes. Colostrum, found in breast milk, fights both viruses and fungi. All these nutrients work together synergistically to strengthen the immune system of the child.

Then, as if all of that were not wonderful enough, researchers now have found that the balance of nutrients and the caloric content of the mother's breast milk will change according to the infant's needs! No wonder the Psalmist observed, *"Out of the mouth of babes and sucklings has thou ordained strength"* (Psalm 8:2 KJV). No manmade formula on the market today could even compare with the design of mother's milk.

However, past the age of three, humans begin to lose rapidly two of the enzymes that are needed to digest milk, namely renin and lactase. Without these enzymes at work, the digestion of milk places a burden on the body, and toxic mucous forms as a by-product of stressed digestion.

In addition, many people cannot digest lactose, the sugar found in milk, and are said to be "lactose intolerant." Digestive problems such as stomachaches, gas, bloating, belching, constipation, or diarrhea can develop. Also, respiratory problems arise from those who are not able to digest other ingredients in milk, such as casein.

A concern is usually voiced when considering whether or not to consume milk and dairy products. People wonder how they will get the calcium they need without milk and dairy products. However, there are many other sources of calcium available. Dark green leafy vegetables, figs, dates, prunes, and raw nuts are excellent sources. The calcium in plant life is more bioavailable, as well.

Dairy Products (Curds and Whey)

The Bible speaks of *curds* or *butter,* depending upon which translation is used. (The New International Version uses *curds* and The King James Version uses *butter.*) We read in Isaiah 7:21,22 that *in that day, a man will keep alive a young cow and two goats. And because of the abundance of milk they give, he will have curds to eat. All who remain in the land will eat curds and honey.*

Curds are solid pieces of milk protein soured or curdled with acid. Whey is the liquid that is poured off after the curds have formed. (Remember "Little Miss Muffet's" food?) In today's world, foods that would be comparable to curds are buttermilk, yogurt, kefir, cottage cheese and other cheeses. Since these dairy products have been fermented, the lactose is easier to digest than in uncultured dairy products.

CHOICES THAT DIMINISH THE BENEFITS OF MILK AND DAIRY PRODUCTS

As with most foods in the modern diet, we have moved far from the freshness of whole, raw milk and milk products. Processing has turned what could be of benefit to mankind into a substance devoid of natural nutritional value.

Pasteurization

Pasteurization, which was originally used for wine, heats milk at 160° Fahrenheit for up to 45 minutes. As was discussed in Chapter Three, enzymes begin to be affected at temperatures above 117° F and are completely destroyed by 130°F. So, pasteurization destroys natural enzymes found in raw milk.

Since enzymes have been destroyed, the other nutrients are not as available to the body. Calcium and folic acid are less likely to be absorbed by the body. Vitamins and minerals are weakened or destroyed, and the protein is altered. Many people are allergic to this altered protein.

The sale of pasteurized milk used to be against the law because it was known to cause so many health problems. If a person chooses to drink animal milk, certified raw milk is the most nutritious choice. Many health food stores have access to sources where it is available.

Homogenization

The process of homogenization breaks the large butterfat globules in milk into tiny ones evenly distributed throughout the liquid. You cannot see the location of the butterfat. I remember as a child, before homogenization came into use, lifting the cap off the milk and licking the butterfat cream that had risen to the top. Then, the milkman began delivering homogenized milk and the cream was no longer there.

One of the main problems with homogenization is that the tiny globules do not bounce through the small bowel as the larger globules in raw milk do. Instead, they pass quickly into the bloodstream, causing a host of cardiovascular problems.

Another danger is that they can cause scarring as they travel through the arteries. This enables cholesterol to attach to the scars and produce arteriosclerosis.

The most healthful animal milk is organic certified raw goat's milk (cow's milk is second). This milk is not only alkaline but it also contains live enzymes making its nutrients more usable by the body.

The next best choice is pasteurized milk that has not been homogenized. The least healthful choice, unfortunately, is the one most people drink—pasteurized and homogenized milk. Most local health food stores can help customers find sources for organic raw milk as some states generally will not allow the sale of milk that has not been pasteurized.

Babes and Sucklings

One of the most detrimental deceptions to sweep this nation in recent years is the false belief that prepared formula is better for babies than mother's breast milk. As a result of this campaign, coupled with our desire for convenience, formula-fed children lack the natural immunity provided by mother's breast milk.

It should be a clue for us that popular formula companies tout the fact that they are "closer to mother's milk" than their competitors. Their aim to be close to mother's milk indicates that mother's milk is the optimum. Processed formula is canned and enriched with synthetic vitamins and minerals, stored in aluminum cans, then warmed to serve. Mother's milk is full of natural essential nutrients served at exactly the right temperature. Man simply cannot, and never will be able to, improve on God.

Poor Choices When Shopping

When shopping for dairy products (curds), there are several factors that should be taken into consideration. One of the most important is the amount of processing the food has undergone.

When choosing cheese, it is best to avoid yellow cheeses because they are not only heavily processed, they have been dyed to add color. Lighter colored cheeses, especially those made from sheep and/or goat's milk, are best. Two popular ones are feta and asiago.

Live culture yogurt has health benefits that pasteurized yogurt does not contain. Always check ingredients' labels of yogurt to see what has been added. You will be amazed to see how many grams of sugar are added, especially if it contains fruit. The best choice is to buy plain live culture yogurt and add your own fruit if you choose to do so.

As discussed in Chapter Three, butter is more healthful than margarine because margarine is a man-made trans-fat that the body does not have the enzymes to digest. However, the ingredients' labels of butter should be checked for chemical additives.

Cruelty to Cattle

I feel I cannot end this section without pointing out how cattle are mistreated on most factory farms. Cattle, noted for being docile animals, have strong attachments to their young. However, the calves of the modern milk cow are taken from them immediately after birth. The reason—the industry tries to keep the cows producing as much milk as possible. Since artificial growth chemicals are used for milk production, the udder of a cow becomes so large it could be damaged if the calf tried to nurse from it. Also, if the bonding that takes place when a calf nurses from its mother were allowed to happen, the mother cow would become quite upset when the calf is removed.

Often with the umbilical cords still attached, female calves are taken to become milk cows and male calves are taken away to be raised for veal or as steers to be slaughtered. In many cases their "milk fed diets" consist of government surplus skim milk with added fat.

With consumers demanding more meat at cheaper prices, the industry has responded to our cries. It has reacted by subjecting docile, "clean" animals to torturous treatment, all so we can overindulge in what should be a special occasion delicacy. What kind of stewards are we for the animals over which God has given us dominion?

II. ANIMALS THAT MOVE ALONG THE GROUND (CREEPING THING)

According to the Bible, *creatures that move along the ground* are not intended for the human diet, therefore those animals will not be considered in the nutritional application of The Creation Diet. The choice of whether or not to eat them is a personal one.

III. WILD ANIMALS

The Bible also strictly condemns eating *wild animals*. Therefore animals in that category will be excluded from the nutritional application of The Creation Diet. Again, the choice of whether or not to eat them is a personal one.

IV. MAN—THE CROWNING WORK OF CREATION

In the words of King David, *"I will praise you because I am fearfully and wonderfully made"* (Psalm 139:14). The human body is one of God's most complex creations.

Fearfully and Wonderfully Made
Each of the 100+ trillion cells that comprise the body is so small it cannot be seen without a microscope, but what occurs inside each cell is amazingly complex. Researchers estimate that the wisdom

found in the cells of one human being exceeds the knowledge that mankind has accumulated collectively to this point in history!

Each one of the cells in the body is a separate entity capable of functioning solely on its own. It moves; it breathes; it digests; it excretes; and it reproduces. However, even though it is perfectly capable of living unto itself, each cell chooses to live for the good of the whole organism—the human body. Scientists do not understand how each cell discerns to work cooperatively with other cells to form and sustain organs and systems. This is one of the marvels of God's crowning work of creation.

The cells that form the 96,000 miles of the **cardiovascular**, or **circulatory system**, cooperate with the cells that comprise the blood, pumping from the heart at a rate of around 100,000 beats every twenty-four hours. During that same time span, the six quarts of blood cells travel 3,000-5,000 times throughout the body, delivering nutrients to organ cells, fighting invaders, and transporting waste for excretion.

The cells cooperate to form another network of vessels, the **lymphatic system**. This system circulates disease-fighting fluids and returns them to the bloodstream.

The cells that form the **respiratory system** cooperate to allow the gas exchange of oxygen inhaled from the air and carbon dioxide removed from the blood and exhaled back into the air.

The 30,000 million cells that form the **nervous system** cooperate to send, receive, and process nerve impulses throughout the body. The brain, a part of this system, only weighs around three pounds, yet every conscious and unconscious activity of the body depends upon its commands.

The cells that comprise the **digestive system** cooperate to transform food into nutrients that build and repair all other cells. They aid also in the removal of solid waste from the system.

The cells that form the **urinary system** cooperate in removing waste from the blood and excreting it as urine. Even though the kidneys are each only the size of a person's ear, they help regulate the pH balance of bodily fluids.

The 100 million cells that form the **immune system** cooperate within varied organ cells. They work together as a unit to protect the body against bacteria, viruses, parasites, fungi, and chain reactions of damaged free radical cells.

The cells that form the **endocrine system** cooperate in producing valuable hormones necessary for bodily functions. These cells alone involve more chemical reactions than all the chemical factories in the world.

The cells that form the bones of the **skeletal system** cooperate to produce the lightweight material (only comprising about one-fifth of our body weight), of extremely hard consistency, needed to support the human frame. These cells help make it possible for the average person to walk some 65,000 miles, or more than 2 ½ times around the earth, in a lifetime. At birth, a newborn baby has over 300 bones, many of which are soft and pliable allowing passage through the birth canal. These soft, pliable bones gradually fuse together to form the 206 hard bones that comprise the adult body.

The cells that form the **muscular system** work together in the following three groups: smooth muscles which control all the automatic or involuntary activity of the body; striated muscles which control deliberate movements and motions; and cardiac muscles, which assist the beating of the heart. The movements of these six hundred muscles use a large amount of the energy formed by the body as food is digested.

The cells that form the **reproductive system** cooperate in allowing a sperm cell to unite with an egg cell to conceive and sustain life until birth. Life, which begins with one cell, divides exponentially as the fetus develops. Inside the gene of each cell is the DNA, or genetic blueprint, that was formed when the traits of an individual's father united with the traits of his or her mother. Because DNA is wound so tightly, a person's DNA is compacted to about the size of an ice cube. However, if it were possible to unwind the DNA in just one person and join it end to end, it would reach from the earth to the sun and back more than four hundred times.

Since each person is uniquely created, the DNA of each person is unique and it carries every morsel of information about that person. It has been estimated that if the intelligence inherent in the DNA of a person could be transcribed, it would fill a thousand books at six hundred pages each.

With all the activity going on in the body every day, all day long, enough heat is generated at any given moment to completely self-destruct. Yet with the body's built-in **cooling system**, we maintain a constant temperature of around 98.6° Fahrenheit. Yes, King David, we are *fearfully and wonderfully made!*

The Secret to Health Can Be Found in the Way God Created Man

Through the story of creation, God showed us the way to health, not only in the sequential order of the days of creation, but also in the way God created man. God has once again taught a lesson within a lesson. Let us focus attention to the account of the creation of Adam as found in Genesis 2:6,7: *. . . but streams came up from the earth and watered the whole surface of the ground—the Lord God formed the man from the dust of the ground and breathed into his nostrils the breath of life, and the man became a living being.*

The Hebrew word used in this verse for *breath* is *neshamah*, meaning "puff (for example, wind); vital breath; divine inspiration, soul, spirit." Considering this, we can see that the following pattern in the creation of man coincides with the concept of The Creation Diet:

Water

Chapter Two dealt in length with the importance of water for the human body. The fact that sixty-five percent of the body is comprised of water gives an idea of how important it is to health. In fact, as was presented in Chapter Two, the blood is 90% water, muscle is 72% water, and the brain is 75% water. Even fat is 15% water, bone is 30% water, and the skin is 71% water.

The dissolving property of water makes it vital to our health. We require water to dissolve the substances we use for food, transport these dissolved nutrients, and carry waste products out of the body. Even a small amount of dehydration causes a disturbance in cellular activity.

Every function of the body depends upon an adequate supply of water. Therefore, it is important that we constantly hydrate our bodies with pure water.

Dust of the Ground

The Lord God formed the man from the dust of the ground

(Genesis 2:7). The importance of plant life that also springs from the ground is detailed in Chapter Three. Virtually all the materials that formed us are found in the soil of the earth. The body is not able to manufacture minerals from other substances within the body, so it must receive them directly, or indirectly, from the soil. Since plants draw their nutrients from the soil, eating plant life—vegetables, seeds (including nuts, whole grains, and legumes), and fruits— enables us to ingest the minerals found in them. The importance of minerals to the chemical balance of the body cannot be overstated.

Also, when we ingest pure, raw plant foods, the live enzymes in them cause the plant cells to be drawn supernaturally to the human cells that need their healing nutrients. As previously stated, in raw organic foods, the forward-spin and reverse-spin of the electrons align to create a burst of pure light. This "body of light" as it is called is able to repair even damaged DNA in a cell. Thus it is possible to break the cycle of disease!

Once again God has given a beautiful foreshadowing of this truth from the Hebrew language. Biblical Hebrew has no vowels but consists only of consonants. To make it pronounceable vowels were later added.

As was mentioned in a previous chapter, the letters (conso-nants) in *owr* (אר), the word for *light,* and in the word for *mouth* (פה), when combined, are the same as the letters in the two words for *heal* (*rapha* רפא or *raphah* רפה). Even the language of the Torah paints a picture that foods with a body of light taken through the mouth will heal. Therefore, as presented in Chapter Three, the ingestion of live enzymes found in pure, raw plant life is a major factor in the difference between health and disease.

Air (Vital Breath)

Air, particularly oxygen, is the single most important nutrient we take into our bodies on a daily basis. In fact, life is not possible without it. This is dealt with extensively in Chapter Two.

The Hebrew meaning of "vital breath" is expressed beautifully, for truly it is vital to our health. Medical professionals confirm that after only four minutes without oxygen our brains sustain damage.

Not only did God show us that the breath was vital, but He even gave us a picture of the importance of breathing deeply. In Genesis

2:7, when God *breathed into his* [Adam's] *nostrils the breath of life,* the Hebrew word used for *breathed* is *naphach*, which literally means "to inflate; to blow hard."

The majority of the gas exchange of oxygen and carbon dioxide takes place in the bottom portion of the lung in the tiny air sacs called the alveoli. Throughout the entire day and night these little alveoli pass oxygen into the blood where it is taken to the heart and pumped throughout the body. The blood brings a waste product (carbon dioxide) from the cells back to the alveoli where it is exhaled through breathing.

The most efficient gas exchange takes place when deep breathing occurs. Moderate exercise is so important because it promotes deep breathing and thus more oxygen intake. The importance of oxygenating the blood through exercise is dealt with in Chapter Two. Moderate or aerobic (with oxygen) exercise promotes the presence of stable oxygen molecules in the body. However, over exercising can produce an anaerobic (without oxygen) state that promotes the presence of unstable oxygen molecules, called free radicals, in the body.

Adam was created with a perfect body, yet even he was given a duty that would ensure he exercised moderately: *The Lord God took the man and put him in the Garden of Eden to work it and take care of it* (Genesis 2:15). In addition, the fact that God gave the example of rest on the seventh day implies that man's consistent activity was foreseen.

I constantly am amazed by the many ways God uses illustrations to convey His message. Once again He has shown us, through His example, that it is important to breathe or "blow hard" the "vital breath" to maintain health.

Soul and Spirit

The story of the last day of creation, as found in Genesis 2:6-7, is the same as the beginning of the first day of creation—it begins and ends with God.

The *neshamah* ("soul" and "spirit" as well as "vital breath") was blown into the nostrils of man. The Creator gave from Himself the light and happiness He desired for mankind to experience continually! He literally inflated us, or brought us to life, by sharing

Himself with us.

After the fall of mankind when sin entered the world, He brought us back to life by once again sharing Himself with us. This time it was by giving His life's blood for us. His final "vital breath" sealed the covenant by which our souls and spirits could be free!

CHOICES THAT DIMINISH THE BENEFITS OF GOD'S PLAN FOR MAN

Even though God has given us the design for living, we do not always follow His pattern. Choices that go against God's plan for health as revealed in the way He created man can be summed up in one word—disobedience. God has shown us again and again how He intends for us to live. We are told in James 4:17 that *to him that knoweth to do good, and doeth it not, to him it is sin.* (King James Version)

Symbolically, we stand in the garden with Adam and Eve. God has provided good and abundant living, which He freely offers to us. Will we choose light and happiness for our souls and spirits? Will we take deep breaths of oxygenated fresh air? Will we hydrate our bodies with pure water? Will we take into our mouths good, life giving foods with a healing body of light? Or will we choose Satan's destructive counterfeits? The choice is ours. What will we do?

SPIRITUAL APPLICATION

For God so loved the world that he gave his one and only Son, that whoever believes in Him should not perish, but have eternal life (John 3:16).

Decorations on Earth

During the writing of The Creation Diet, I awakened in the wee hours one morning reflecting on God's beautiful world. As I lay in bed, I pictured tranquil lakes and rolling ocean waves, majestic mountains, pristine forests, and lush green fields. I envisioned animals peacefully grazing together, and I began thanking God for the beautiful world He created.

Then a thought came into my mind and I prayed, "Lord, You

constructed a wonderful, beautiful world. However, it is as though You felt in Your heart that the world would not be complete without each individual person You create."

Suddenly, it occurred to me that the word, *world,* in John 3:16 might have multiple meanings. In the darkness I got up and hurried into my little study to look up the meaning of *world* in the Greek dictionary. What I found made me weep as I realized the depth of God's love!

In the Greek language of John 3:16, *world* is *kosmos*, and it has both a broad and a narrow meaning. In the broad sense it means "an orderly arrangement," as in the orderly way in which God created the world. In the narrow sense, it means "decoration."

God had, through orderly arrangement, created a wonderful, beautiful, perfect world. However, as wonderful and beautiful and perfect as the world was, God did not consider it complete until He carefully created "decorations" for His world. These "decorations" are every person God uniquely creates in His image and likeness! Each of us is an object of God's love, created to decorate His world. Each "decoration" is completely different from any other, but God loves each "decoration" equally.

I greatly admire people who are interior decorators, for I am not gifted particularly in that area. However, even though the different homes in which we have lived throughout our married life have not been fancy, they have been "homey." The things with which we have chosen to decorate our home are not necessarily esthetically beautiful, but they are meaningful to us. These treasures include things such as the shadowboxes that hold memories of when our daughters were babies; pictures embroidered or painted by friends; a stained-glass flower crafted by a friend; collages of family portraits; favorite sayings or mottoes; and family treasures that have been passed down through generations.

A person walking into our home might not think these decorations are pretty, but they are things that we treasure and things that make our house a home. Each one has a special place and a special purpose, and each one makes our home complete.

The same is true of God. Each "decoration" He creates has a special place and a special purpose in this world. We are created uniquely by God and placed in this world because He loves us. We are not mass-produced! God felt that His world would be incomplete without any one of us. Do you comprehend how wonderful that is?

It is humbling to realize that God, the Creator of the universe, chose to create each of us as a decoration for His world. The fact that He would not feel complete without any one of us should be a life changing revelation!

Decorations in Heaven

It is even more humbling to realize that not only does God have a special place for us in this world, He has prepared a special place for each of His decorations in heaven. However, there is something quite different that we must consider at this point.

We did not have a choice about coming into this world. Out of God's love He created us and placed us here. However, we do have a choice about whether or not we will accept God's provision for the world to come. This is where the beauty of John 3:16 comes into full view.

God placed the first perfect "decorations," Adam and Eve, in a perfect world. However, when they chose to believe a lie of Satan and disobey God, sin entered into them and into God's perfect world.

The account of this deception can be found in Genesis 3:1-24. Up until that time, Adam and Eve had known only good. However, when they ate of *the tree of the knowledge of good and evil,* which God specifically had forbidden in Genesis 2:17, they chose to partake of evil. Evil entered into them, became a part of their nature, and they no longer were perfect. The evil that entered into the first man and woman then was passed on to each succeeding generation.

King David made reference to this in Psalm 51:5 when he declared, *"Surely I was sinful at birth, sinful from the time my mother conceived me."* Each person born since the original sin entered into the world is born in the state or condition of sin.

Drastic conditions require drastic measures, and our loving Creator did what was necessary to rectify the damage that had been done. Since the beginning chapter of The Creation Diet, it has been shown that in God's plan *the life is in* the *blood* (Leviticus 17:11). Although there are many applications of this principle throughout scripture, one of the most poignant is in the concept of the system of the blood sacrifice.

The Perfect Sacrifice

God allowed the life of an animal to be substituted for the life of an individual. This great act of mercy toward mankind was established immediately after Adam and Eve sinned. Instead of requiring their human lives, we are told in Genesis 3:21 that *the Lord God made garments of skin for Adam and his wife and clothed them.* The Hebrew word for *clothed* is *labash* meaning "to wrap around." The life of an animal was given in order that Adam and Eve might be "wrapped around" by God—a foreshadowing of things to come.

Earlier in this chapter, the correlation between the requirements of the Passover lamb and the fulfillment by Jesus was presented. After the original Passover, a sacrificial system for the nation of Israel was established. In this system, the blood of a sacrificial animal was poured on the altar, representing that the life of an individual was being laid on the altar, in sacrifice and repentance for sin.

However, God knew that this system was temporary. The Tabernacle and Temple in which to make the sacrifices would not always exist. One day it would be necessary for God to give His own life's blood to restore His decorations to the original condition He intended for them. We are told in scripture that *God is spirit* (John 4:24). So, how could a Spirit die in order for His blood to become the substitutionary sacrifice for our sins?

In an unprecedented act of love and mercy, God willingly came to earth in the form of one of His decorations. God came to earth in bodily form through Jesus Christ, the Son. He became like us so that we could become like Him. Philippians 2:5-8 records,

> *Your attitude should be the same as that of Christ Jesus: Who, being in very nature God, did not consider equality with God something to be grasped, but made himself nothing, taking the very nature of a servant, being made in human likeness. And being found in appearance as a man, he humbled himself and became obedient to death— even death on a cross.*

Through His death on the cross, Jesus became the final blood sacrifice for sin and thereby fulfilled the sacrificial system. The verses in Hebrews 9:1-28 paint a beautiful description of the earthly Tabernacle and its contents (from which the Temple was later designed). This passage illustrates how the priests and the high priest offered sacrifices in the Tabernacle, and later in the Temple. The writer of Hebrews explains that the earthly Tabernacle was based on a heavenly one, not made with human hands. These beautiful verses cite that sacrifices had to be made continually by the priests.

However, at His death, Jesus became the eternal High Priest. His blood took the place of the blood of animals for all time to come. Then, He entered one time into the heavenly Holy of Holies to present His blood as the completion of the sacrificial system.

We are told the following in excerpts from Hebrews 10:1-11:

> *The law is only a shadow of the good things that are coming—not the realities themselves. For this reason it can never, by the same sacrifices repeated endlessly year after year, make perfect those who draw near to worship. If it could, would they not have stopped being offered? For the worshipers would have been cleansed once for all, and would no longer have felt guilty for their sins. But those sacrifices are an annual reminder of sins, because it is impossible for the blood of bulls and goats to take away sins. Therefore, when Christ came into the world, he said: "Sacrifices and offerings you did not desire, but a body you prepared for me; with burnt offerings and sin offerings you were not pleased." Then I said, "Here I am—it is written about me in the scroll—I have come to do your will, O God." . . . And by that will, we have been made holy through the sacrifice of the body of Jesus Christ once for all. Day after day every priest stands and performs his religious duties, again and again he offers the same sacrifices, which can never take away sins. But when this priest had offered for all time one sacrifice*

for sins, he sat down at the right hand of God.

God Himself came to earth in the bodily form of Jesus, the promised Messiah, and gave His own blood as the sacrifice for our sins—once and for all, forever and ever, Amen! Those who accept what God has done and receive this eternal gift are assured everlasting life in His beautiful heaven, as a perfect "decoration" loved by God.

Yes, God did so love the world, in the broad and the narrow sense, *that he gave his one and only Son, that whoever believes in Him should not perish, but have eternal life* (John 3:16).

Dear God, Creator of Heaven and Earth,
I bow in humility before You. I cannot comprehend Your intelligence that could think of every detail of creation. I cannot comprehend Your power that could bring into existence every detail of creation. I cannot comprehend Your grace that caused You to create me as a special decoration in Your world. But most of all, I cannot comprehend Your love that compelled You to come to earth as the final and ultimate sacrifice for my sin. I simply say, "Thank You!"
In the name of the Lamb of God I pray, Amen.

MEMORY VERSE FOR CHAPTER SIX:
For God so loved the world that he gave his one and only Son, that whoever believes in Him should not perish, but have eternal life (John 3:16).

ASSIGNMENT(S) FOR CHAPTER SIX:

1. Limit animal products. **Eat red meat of *livestock* *(cattle)* sparingly**. Find unadulterated sources for the meat.

2. **One serving of plain yogurt, kefir, butter, or natural cheese, cottage cheese,** or **buttermil**k (all of which are similar to the biblical *curds*) may be consumed **daily**. The most healthful sources are unpasteurized and unhomogenized. Consumption of liquid goat's milk and cow's milk should be limited, and should come from organic, certified, raw sources. An alternative to

animal milk is vegetable milk. Good sources include rice, almond, and natural non-hybrid soy milk.

3. Commit to **moderate exercise** at least **five days per week.**

DEVOTIONAL FOR CHAPTER SIX

Day One

Scripture Reading: Psalm 50:1-15

Verse of the Day: . . .*for every animal of the forest is mine, and the cattle on a thousand hills* (Psalm 50:10).

When I was a child, my family traveled often to the mountains of North Carolina where my grandmother was raised. I remember being fascinated by the large herds of cattle we saw grazing in mountain pastures.

Today's related verse gives me great comfort. It helps me realize that just as God owns everything in this world, including *the cattle on a thousand hills,* certainly He has the resources to take care of all my needs. He also has the desire to do so.

We are assured in Philippians 4:19 that. . . *my God will meet all your needs according to his glorious riches in Christ Jesus.* The first part of that verse is thrilling. Just knowing that God will supply all my needs is wonderful. But, the verse does not end there. God not only promises to supply all my needs, He promises to do so according to His riches in glory. How rich is God?

As Psalm 50 clearly states, He owns everything on the earth and in heaven. All things belong to Him. His resources are unlimited. That is as rich as you can get.

Therefore, whenever we have a need, we can rest assured that God will fill that need from His treasure of unlimited supplies. His Word promises us so.

The fact that God will supply our needs is a wonderful realization. The fact that He will do so according to His riches in glory is an even more astounding awareness. However, the most wonderful realization of all is the way in which He chooses to supply our needs through *Christ Jesus*. Those who have come into a relationship with God through His Son, Jesus Christ, never have to worry about anything. Every need will be met—abundantly, miraculously, lovingly.

What are we to do in response? The answer is found in Psalm 50:14,15. We are to trust God to meet every need. As the Psalmist suggests, we are to *call upon* God. Then, when He supplies our needs as He has promised, we are to *sacrifice thank offerings to God. . . fulfill vows to the Most High...* and *honor* Him.

I once heard the story of a seminary that needed a large sum of money in order to remain open. The president prayed in faith that since God owned *the cattle on a thousand hills,* He would provide what the school needed. Unknowingly, a wealthy cattle rancher felt led to make a large donation in the exact amount the school needed. As a member of the Board of Trustees handed the cattleman's check to the seminary president, he smiled and said, "I think God just sold some of those cows."

Application:

1) Do you have a need in your life that seems overwhelming? Pray the prayer of faith.
2) Be careful to thank God and glorify Him when He supplies your need.

PRAY and thank God in advance for the way(s) He will choose to answer your prayer.

DEVOTIONAL FOR CHAPTER SIX

Day Two

Scripture Reading: Psalm 23:1-6

Verse of the Day: *We all, like sheep, have gone astray, each of us has turned to his own way; and the Lord has laid on him the iniquity of us all* (Isaiah 53:6).

Throughout the Bible, we are compared to sheep (a part of the cattle family), and God is compared to our Shepherd. The following are characteristics of sheep verified through familiar verses taken from the King James Version of Psalm 23:

Sheep are considered unintelligent. Without supervision, sheep often make poor choices. All their needs have to be met by the shepherd or they will die: *The Lord is my Shepherd; I shall not want* (v.1).

Sheep have a tendency to keep moving, to the point of exhaustion. The shepherd plans time for his sheep to rest: *He maketh me to lie down in green pastures. . .* (v.2).

Sheep often sink rather than swim since their wet fleece weighs them down. They must be kept away from swift water when they are thirsty to prevent possible drowning: *. . . He leadeth me beside the still waters* (v.2).

Sheep are lost easily. If they stray from the shepherd, they wander away from the flock, becoming lost and alone: *. . . He leadeth me in the paths of righteousness for His name's sake* (v.3).

Sheep are defenseless. Without the shepherd's protection, they are easy prey for predators: *Yea, though I walk through the valley of the shadow of death, I will fear no evil for Thou art with me; Thy rod and Thy staff they comfort me* (v.4).

Sheep do not know the difference between what is good for them and what is harmful. While grazing, they will eat poisonous herbs if the shepherd does not lead them to safe pastures or pluck the poisonous herbs from fertile pastures: *Thou preparest a table before me in the presence of mine enemies. . .* (v.5).

Sheep are almost blind. They cannot see very far in front of them. As a result, they run head on into things that hurt them. They depend on the shepherd to apply healing oils and balms to their wounds: *. . . Thou anointest my head with oil. . .* (v.5).

Sheep are thirsty after a long day. A cup of cool water straight from the Shepherd's hand soothes their dry, parched throats: *. . . my cup runneth over* (v.5).

Sheep form a strong attachment to their shepherd. They have faith that he will take care of their needs: *Surely goodness and mercy shall follow me all the days of my life: and I will dwell in the house of the Lord forever* (v.6).

Being a shepherd requires total commitment to the sheep. Shepherds often have lost their lives while caring for the needs of their sheep. That is what happened to our good Shepherd. Because of His death, *I will dwell in the house of the Lord forever.*

Application:
1) The Good Shepherd cares tenderly for you. Have you entered into His fold?

PRAY and thank The Good Shepherd for dying so that you could live.

DEVOTIONAL FOR CHAPTER SIX

Day Three

Scripture Reading: Exodus 4:1-17

Verse of the Day: *The Lord said, "Throw it on the ground." Moses threw it on the ground and it became a snake, and he ran from it* (Exodus 4:3).

Moses had been a shepherd for forty years in the wilderness of Midian. His shepherd's rod had been an important part of his own protection, as well as the protection of his flock. No doubt he had used it on many occasions to fight off dangerous animals, or possibly even other people trying to steal his sheep. He depended on this rod, which gave him a sense of security.

Therefore, God had Moses throw his "security" to the ground. God was teaching early on that He would be Moses' security, not a piece of wood. Notice that God did not ask that he gently lay it down; he had to *throw* it down. Moses was required to rid himself of it quickly in a deliberate act of obedience. Perhaps this was one of the most difficult tasks God could have asked Moses to do.

As soon as Moses obeyed God, the true nature of Moses' dependence on the rod was revealed. The shepherd's rod became a serpent, the biblical picture of Satan, *that ancient serpent, who is the devil, or Satan...* (Revelation 20:2).

Nothing was inherently wrong with the rod itself, for it was only a piece of wood. However, God knew that anyone or anything that usurped Moses' dependence upon Him was wrong.

The very thing that Moses had once clung to with all his might was now the thing from which he ran. The object that had kept him from fear now brought him fear. Ironically, he now ran for protection from what had been his protection.

God then told Moses to pick up the serpent. In another deliberate act of faithful obedience (and to me, picking up a snake required a lot of faith) he did as God asked, and the serpent was transformed back into a shepherd's rod. It was no longer the rod of Moses. It was now the rod of God. This rod was used to confound Pharaoh's magicians, to part the Red Sea, and to lead hundreds of thousands of Israelites through the wilderness. All of this was possible because Moses was willing to let go and let God control his life.

One of the most powerful songs I have ever heard is "Moses" by Ken Medema. The closing lines express the following:

> *What do you hold in your hand today?*
> *To what or to whom are you bound?*
> *Are you willing to give it to God right now?*
> *Give it up, let it go, throw it down!*

Application:

1) Survey your life. Is there anything to whom or to which you are holding more tightly than God?
2) If so, cast it down. With God's help, pick it up again in the proper perspective.

PRAY and ask God to help you grow in your total dependence upon Him.

DEVOTIONAL FOR CHAPTER SIX

Day Four

Scripture Reading: Daniel 6:1-28

Verse of the Day: *Be sure of this: The wicked will not go unpunished, but those who are righteous will go free* (Proverbs 11:21).

As a teenager, Daniel was among the brightest and best Jewish people who were taken captive into Babylon. Daniel was a young man who was righteous (Ezekiel 14:14) and wise (Ezekiel 28:3). However, his most outstanding characteristic is that he appears to have been committed totally to God. He always stood for his convictions.

By the time of the events in today's passage, Daniel was over eighty years old. During his time in Babylon, he had served under three kings, the last being Darius. King Darius planned to reorganize Babylon into 129 provinces with three presidents. Daniel was appointed as a president because of his wisdom and integrity.

King Darius became so impressed with Daniel, he considered placing him above the other two presidents. The other presidents became so jealous, they tricked King Darius into signing a thirty-day decree stating that all prayer during that time period had to be directed to him as king. The two presidents felt sure Daniel would break the decree, and he did.

He continued to face Jerusalem and pray to the God of Israel three times a day. The result was that King Darius sorrowfully had to adhere to his edict, thus casting Daniel into a pit with hungry lions.

The next morning he rushed to the pit and had the capstone removed. King Darius found that God had sent an angel to shut the mouths of the lions. The king then issued a new decree ordering all the citizens in his kingdom to consider worshipping the true God.

Standing up for our commitment to God is not always easy, but always rewarding. Most of the time the situations in which we are placed for Him cause us more "alarm" than "harm." Daniel was willing to stand for his convictions no matter the cost. In the words of an old song, are we willing to "Dare to be a Daniel?"

Application:

1) Are those around you able to look at your life and recognize your commitment to God?
2) In what ways do you show your commitment? In what ways do you not?
3) Determine to take one step toward being a more public example of God's love.

PRAY and ask God to give you courage to stand up for your convictions like Daniel.

DEVOTIONAL FOR CHAPTER SIX

Day Five

Scripture Reading: Luke 10:1-21

Verse of the Day: *I am sending you out like sheep among wolves. Therefore be as shrewd as snakes and as innocent as doves* (Matthew 10:16).

The time had come for Jesus to make His final journey to Jerusalem. This is the journey that would end His life. Because the threats of impending death had become so strong, Jesus sent His followers as forerunners. Their mission was to prepare the way and announce His coming to the villages along the way.

In Luke 9:1-6, Jesus sent the twelve apostles on a similar mission from Northern Galilee. Now He was sending seventy other followers by pairs.

Jesus first instructed them to pray for more laborers. This is an obvious answer to spreading the gospel around the world, yet it is one that is often ignored. Many believers feel that they are overworked and overburdened, yet they fail to pray for more laborers.

Secondly, the followers were sent to spread the gospel fully aware of the fact that they would face persecution. In a real sense, Jesus was preparing them for the coming persecution of the church that would follow His death. He told them that He was sending them forth *like lambs among wolves* (Luke 10:3).

Wolves are known as predators. They are flesh-eating animals that often travel in packs. Wolves are enemies of livestock farmers. A pack of wolves can attack an entire herd of cows or sheep. Jesus' followers well understood this metaphor. Like lambs among wolves, their lives would be in danger. Yet, they were to remain faithful to the mission.

Luke 10:17-21 contains the reports of the seventy missionaries. They returned with great joy, amazed at the power they had experienced. Even devils were subject to them. Jesus saw the danger in their astonishment. He quickly turned their attention away from what they had done to what God had done for them. He moved the emphasis away from their authority over the devils to the fact that their names were written in heaven. Jesus knew that pride is one of the "wolves" that devours His sheep.

This section concludes with a verse that warms my heart. We read in Luke 10:21, that *in that hour Jesus rejoiced in Spirit.* (KJV). The Greek word used here for *rejoiced* is *agalliao,* and literally it means "to jump for joy." Can you visualize this? Our Savior was so proud of His students He literally jumped for joy.

I often hear people say they want to please God, but they do not know how. The key to pleasing God is found in making sure your name is written in heaven.

Application:

1) Is your name written in heaven? If so, have you accepted His commission?

PRAY and thank God for His provision for you. Ask Him to help you be faithful to Him even in the midst of persecution.

DEVOTIONAL FOR CHAPTER SIX

Day Six

Scripture Reading: Psalm 8:1-9; Hebrews 2:6-9

Verse of the Day: *And being found in appearance as a man, he* *humbled himself and became obedient to death—even death on a cross!* (Philippians 2:8)

Today's scripture reading is a further confirmation of the creation narrative. God prepared a beautiful, wonderful world and then placed man in the world. Man's mission was to tend God's creations and have dominion over them.

Both passages state that man was made a little lower than the angels. From the dawn of the world man was considered such a special creation, he was only a little lower than the angels. Both passages confirm that man was crowned with honor and glory.

Then, man chose to sin and symbolically the crown fell from his head to the dust. God longed for man to return to what he had been created to be originally. There was only one way mankind could regain his crown of honor and glory.

In Hebrews 2:9, we are told how God accomplished this: *But we see Jesus, who was made a little lower than the angels, now crowned with glory and honor because he suffered death, so that by the grace of God he might taste death for everyone.*

At a climactic point in history God Himself came down to earth through Jesus, the physical manifestation of the Godhead. The Creator took on the form of the created. He, Who had created the angels, was suddenly made a little lower than the angels. In an unprecedented act of mercy and grace, Jesus came to earth for the purpose of suffering death on our behalves.

Can we even fathom what that really means? At His death, it is as if Jesus took the crown of glory and honor from the dust and offered to place it on the head of *everyone* (Hebrews 2:9) who would accept it. We are told in scripture that those who choose to accept His gift will one day judge the angels (I Corinthians 6:3,4).

I often wish I could have something of great value to give to God for all He has done for me. One day a thought came to me that filled my heart with joy. I pictured myself kneeling in His presence and lovingly placing my crown at His feet. Then I realized something profound. If it were not for Him I would not even have a crown to present. It really belongs to Him anyway.

Application:

1) Where is your crown? Is it still in the dust, or have you allowed Jesus to place it back on your head?
2) If you have, thank Him for providing the way for you to regain glory and honor. If you have not, search your heart to see what is keeping you from doing so.

PRAY and thank Jesus for tasting death on your behalf.

DEVOTIONAL FOR CHAPTER SIX

Day Seven

Scripture Reading: John 1:19-39

Verse(s) of the Day: *For you know that it was not with perishable things such as silver or gold that you were redeemed. . . but with the precious blood of Christ, a lamb without blemish or defect"* (I Peter 1:18,19).

What is your earliest childhood memory? What feeling does it evoke when you think about it? My earliest memory is a decal of a little lamb that was on my crib. When I was five years old, my sister was born, and the crib became hers.

My sister was born with serious physical problems. Many times when I was a child, I stood and watched her sleep. I loved her so much, and whenever I felt worried about her illness, looking at the little lamb on the crib comforted me. I somehow felt the lamb was watching over my baby sister. Even now as I think of it, I feel safe and secure.

Three years later, when I was eight years old, I opened my heart to the only Lamb who could truly offer security. Even at that young age, I understood that I was a sinner and that God had provided the answer for my salvation.

In today's scripture reading, John was questioned about being the promised Messiah. He declared that he was not, but his mission was to prepare the way for the Promised One. The next day, John saw Jesus coming toward him. Immediately recognizing Him, John exclaimed, *"Look, the Lamb of God, who takes away the sin of the world!"* (John 1:29)

On this earth, we may never comprehend fully the depth of God's love. He loved each of us so much, He died in place of us so that we could live. His death fulfilled the sacrificial system given by God in the Torah. His death, burial, and resurrection fulfilled each feast and festival of Israel. His death was the means by which we could enter into covenant with God. His death provided direct access into the spiritual Holy of Holies where we could experience the presence of God. His death gave us life.

In time, my baby sister recovered from her illness and the crib was given away. However, I will never forget standing and looking at the lamb on the crib. And, praise God, I will never forget standing and looking through scripture at **the** Lamb on the cross.

Lamb of God—Son of Man, Jesus the one and only *who takes away the sin of the world.* To God be the glory!

Application:

1) When was the first time you were told about the Lamb of God? What was your response?
2) In what ways does the Lamb provide for you a sense of security?

PRAY and thank God for providing the means through which you can be saved from your sins. Thank Him for the way(s) the Lamb provides a sense of security for you.

CHAPTER SEVEN

BIBLICAL APPLICATION

The Seventh Day of the Creation Week

(Genesis 2:1-3)

1 Thus the heavens and the earth were completed in all their vast array. 2 By the seventh day God had finished the work he had been doing; so on the seventh day he rested from all his work. 3 And God blessed the seventh day and made it holy, because on it he rested from all the work of creating that he had done.

REST, HOLINESS, AND JOY

Thus the heavens and the earth were completed. . . (Genesis 2:1). A literal rendering of this phrase is "And finished were the heavens and the earth," with the emphasis on the verb "finished." The Hebrew word for "finished" is *kalah* meaning "to end; to be finished; to complete." The word *kalah* carries with it both the connotations of cessation and perfection.

The newly created world was an orderly and beautiful cosmos, filled with teeming plant and animal life and decorated with a man and woman created in God's own image. He had declared everything to be *very good* (Genesis 1:31). All of creation *in all their vast array* (Genesis 2:1) stood at attention for the Creator, like a troop of soldiers arranged in marching order. He had created them, and now their purpose was to glorify Him.

When God created each form of plant and animal life, He also blessed them with the ability to propagate their species. His work of creation was complete and it was perfect in every way: *By the seventh day God had finished the work he had been doing. . .* (Genesis 2:2a).

This does not mean that God was still creating on the seventh day, for clearly scripture shows that man and woman—the final acts of creation—were created before the close of the sixth day (Genesis 1:31). The rabbinical teaching is that God, who knows each exact moment of time, began the seventh day "to a hair's breath" close to the end of the sixth day. In fact, the Midrash, a collection of Jewish commentaries, has an interesting perspective on the situation. It compares the beginning of the seventh day to a man who raises a hammer while it is still day and in the split second before he brings it down to strike an anvil, it has officially become night.

This is confirmed further in the next phrase of Genesis 2:2 which states that *on the seventh day he rested from all his work.* From the Hebrew word for *rest (shabath)* we derive the word "Sabbath." *Shabath* means "to repose, to desist (stop, cease from exertion)" and by implication "to keep Sabbath, to celebrate." God ceased the work of creation; He assumed the posture of quiet rest; He celebrated the goodness of His completed world.

I remember well the first moments following the birth of each of our daughters. After several hours of "labor," our children were born. The time had come to rest from my labor and to celebrate. It was truly a spiritual experience.

One of my happiest memories is the feeling I experienced when I beheld those beautiful creations. I observed every detail of their tiny beings, overwhelmed with emotion. There in my arms was a part of my beloved husband and me. The labor had ceased and the long awaited event had taken place, and it was very good.

With the completion of creation, God observed every tiny detail of His new beings, overwhelmed with emotion. There in His arms was a part of Himself. The labor had ceased and the long awaited event had taken place, . . . *and it was very good. . .* (Genesis 1:31).

The narrative of the creation week continues with the words

"And God blessed the seventh day". . . (Genesis 2:3). God previously had blessed the fish and fowl created on the fifth day and man and woman created on the sixth day. In this passage, He blesses the seventh day itself. This is the first account of an actual period of time receiving a blessing. On all other days, the creations were the beneficiaries of His blessing.

By blessing the seventh day, God declared it to be a special object of His divine favor. In turn, it was to be a day of blessing for His creations. By His design both God and man receive a blessing from the Sabbath.

In addition to blessing the seventh day, God also *made it holy,* in the King James Version, *sanctified* it (Genesis 2:3). The Hebrew word for *sanctify* is *qadash* meaning "to be, make, pronounce or observe as clean (ceremonially and morally); consecrate, dedicate, hallow, to be or keep holy." The seventh day was a "clean" day that was to be dedicated and observed as a holy day.

The Sabbath, which was the only day God assigned a name, conveys a profound meaning. Through it, God showed us an example of how to live happy and healthy lives.

We are told elsewhere in scripture that God never rests, nor needs to rest. The Psalmist wrote in Psalm 121:3,4, that. . . *he who watches over you will not slumber; indeed, he who watches over Israel will neither slumber nor sleep."* Also, we read in Isaiah 40:28, *"Do you not know? Have you not heard? The Lord is the everlasting God, the Creator of the ends of the earth. He will not grow tired or weary, and his understanding no one can fathom."*

God's example of rest teaches us to observe the Sabbath as a holy day. The closing phrase of Genesis 2:3 expresses why it was deemed holy: God *made it holy, because on it he rested from all the work of creating that he had done.*

Following God's Example

Scripture confirms that God never has the need to rest, therefore we must delve deeper into Genesis 2:1-3 to see what His day of rest means to us. Let us consider again the Hebrew words for *rest* and *sanctify.* Since *rest* means "to repose, to desist (stop, cease from exertion); to keep Sabbath, to celebrate" and *sanctify* means "to be, make, pronounce or observe as clean (ceremonially and morally);

consecrate, dedicate, hallow, to be or keep holy," there must be a lesson that benefits our lives.

Inherent in God's resting and sanctification of the seventh day we find three major elements. God's intention was that the Sabbath be a day of rest, a day set aside for holiness, and a day of celebration and joy.

To this day, Jewish people make the three elements modeled in this passage a part of Sabbath observances. From sundown on Friday until sundown on Saturday, rest, holiness, and joy characterize the Sabbath celebration in observant Jewish homes.

Rest: Observant Jews do not work on the Sabbath, but prepare in advance for the activities of the day. The main focus of their rest is to enjoy relaxation. It is a time for restful activities such as napping or taking a walk. In Israel, many Jewish people are allowed to go home from their jobs early on Friday before the Sabbath begins.

Holiness: Special blessings and ceremonies accompany the Sabbath meal. In addition to personal worship of God, it is a time for corporate worship at the synagogue. The Friday evening service is brief so the people can return home for the Sabbath meal. The Saturday morning service includes reading from the Torah and the Haftarah which are selections from the biblical books of the prophets. The Torah is divided into fifty-two divisions in order that one may be read weekly. The Haftarah selections refer to the Torah reading for that day.

Joy: The joy of the Sabbath is heightened by the time enjoyed with family and friends. Singing and special ceremonies accompany the Sabbath dinner. Fun, laughter, and happy times mark it as a true celebration.

The story is told that the Rabbi Yisrael Meir HaCohen once met a fellow Jew who chose to work rather than to observe the Sabbath. The rabbi simply took the man's hand between his own hands and wept, saying, "Shabbat, Shabbat," ("Sabbath, Sabbath"). After a few moments, the other man broke into weeping also. From that time on, the worker was found in the synagogue every Sabbath.

The Sabbath in Bible Times

The Bible does not mention whether or not the Patriarchs

observed the Sabbath, however, rabbinical teachings say that they did. As close as their relationship was with God, Adam and Eve would have been made aware of its importance.

The earliest reference to the Sabbath actually being explained is in the sixteenth chapter of Exodus. While the children of Israel were in the wilderness, God promised to provide six days worth of a bread-like substance, called manna, to be gathered each morning. However, on the sixth day, they were to gather twice as much to provide for their needs on the seventh day.

Moses then told them, ". . . *This is what the Lord commanded: 'Tomorrow is to be a day of rest, a holy Sabbath to the Lord. So bake what you want to bake and boil what you want to boil. Save whatever is left and keep it until morning'"* (Exodus 16:23).

Some of the people did not obey and went to gather manna on the Sabbath, but there was none. Moses scolded, *"Bear in mind that the Lord has given you the Sabbath; that is why on the sixth day he gives you bread for two days. Everyone is to stay where he is on the seventh day; no one is to go out."* So the people rested on the seventh day (Exodus 16:29,30).

Approximately three weeks later, the Ten Commandments were given to the nation of Israel at Mt. Sinai. The fourth commandment declared that the Sabbath was to be holy. Approximately thirty percent of the instructions in the Ten Commandments, or 98 of the 322 words relate to keeping the Sabbath holy.

> *Remember the Sabbath day by keeping it holy. Six days you shall labor and do all your work, but the seventh day is a Sabbath to the Lord your God. On it you shall not do any work, neither you, nor your son or daughter, nor your manservant or maidservant, nor your animals, nor the alien within your gates. For in six days the Lord made the heavens and the earth, the sea, and all that is in them, but he rested on the seventh day. Therefore, the Lord blessed the Sabbath day and made it holy* (Exodus 20:8-11).

In additional commandments given in the Torah, the Israelites were instructed to also observe a Sabbatical year. The Creator knew that even the land, which supported plant life, animals and man, would need time to rest and replenish.

> *For six years you are to sow your fields and harvest*
> *the crops, but during the seventh year let the land lie*
> *unplowed and unused. Then the poor among your*
> *people may get food from it, and the wild animals*
> *may eat what they leave. Do the same with your*
> *vineyard and your olive grove. . .* (Exodus 23:10,11).

During this Sabbatical year, poor people and field animals were welcome to any spontaneous produce that grew.

In addition, during this time, to keep poverty out of the nation of Israel, creditors were commanded to release their debtors from financial burdens.

> *At the end of every seven years you must cancel debts.*
> *This is how it is to be done: Every creditor shall*
> *cancel the loan he has made to his fellow Israelite. He*
> *shall not require payment from his fellow Israelite or*
> *brother, because the Lord's time for canceling debts*
> *has been proclaimed* (Deuteronomy 15:1,2).

The Sabbath was to be a sign of the covenant between God and Israel (Exodus 31:16). Paul clearly states that through the New Covenant sealed by the blood of Jesus, Christians are grafted into the *olive tree,* the nation of Israel (Romans 11:17). Therefore, Christians also are expected to observe the Sabbath.

The Change from the Sabbath to the Lord's Day

Various scriptures refer to the fact that Jesus, and later the early church, observed the Sabbath. However, in 132 A.D., Simon Bar-Kochba led a revolt against the Romans in which tens of thousands of men and women were killed or sold into slavery. As a result, Jews were forbidden to enter Jerusalem, and the name of the whole region was changed to Palestine. It became increasingly dangerous to be associated with the Jews, so Christians began to worship on Sunday rather than on Saturday.

Later, the Church of Rome issued the following statement:

Christians shall not Judaize and be idle on Saturday, the Sabbath, but shall work on that day; but the Lord's day [Sunday] they shall honor, and as being Christians, shall if possible, do no work on that day. If, however, they are found Judaizing, they shall be shut out from Christ.

(What an atrocious statement that those who observed the true Sabbath would be "shut out from Christ"!)

It is stated in the Catholic Encyclopedia that "Sunday observance is from when the Catholic Church transferred the solemnity from Saturday to Sunday." Therefore, the concept of the Sabbath and the Lord's Day converged and Christians worldwide began to celebrate a "Sunday Sabbath."

It is important to note that the change from the Sabbath (Saturday) to the Lord's Day (Sunday) was a man-made decision in the face of persecution. The change is not sanctioned anywhere in scripture. However, we have "inherited" this change from Saturday to Sunday. Therefore, it should be observed with the same intensity as the true Sabbath.

The Sabbath was Made for Man

Most people, if they observe the Sabbath at all, see it merely as a day to slow down rather than to rest. God intended that man, created in His image, follow His example and rest one day a week.

On one end of the spectrum are those who do not observe a Sabbath and work seven days a week. On the other end of the spectrum are those who have laden the Sabbath with unending rules regarding what *rest* means.

God's intention was that man would observe a weekly Sabbath in order to be restored—spirit, soul and body. In fact, "restore" comes from the same root word as *rest*. In the Bible there is one positive or "do" commandment and one negative or "do not" commandment associated with the Sabbath.

The "do" is found in Leviticus 23:3. The Sabbath was to be *a day of sacred assembly* when people gathered to worship God.

While it is true that we can worship God alone and that we can worship Him every day of the week, it is true also that God ordained one day a week to unite in corporate worship.

I have observed something significant when enjoying a bonfire while on youth retreats or other gatherings. The logs will burn as long as they are in a pile with other logs. However, if one falls away from the fire, or is removed for some reason, it soon loses its fire. Like the logs of a bonfire, corporate worship helps to ignite and sustain the fire of our passion for God.

The "do not" of the Sabbath is found in various places throughout the Torah, and it simply admonishes "*. . . you shall not do any work. . .* " (Exodus 20:10). In fact, working on the Sabbath carried the same punishment as murder. In Exodus 31:15 we read, "*. . . Whoever does any work on the Sabbath day must be put to death.*" This proves how seriously God views observing a day of rest.

The Sabbath is an Unending Celebration

Each day of creation had an ending. The words, "*And the evening and the morning were the (first v.5, second v.8, third v.13, fourth v.19, fifth v.23, sixth v.31) day*[s]" denote this. However, there is no ending recorded for the seventh day. The verses regarding the Sabbath in Genesis 2:1-3 do not mention the completion of that day. They end with God blessing the Sabbath because it was the day He rested.

There is a significant reason for this—the Sabbath is unending. The nation of Israel was instructed to observe the Sabbath weekly. The rest, holiness, and joy associated with the weekly Sabbath will find fulfillment when Jesus comes to earth again and establishes His reign on earth and the ultimate fulfillment in heaven. During that time the world will live in complete harmony and peace. The eleventh chapter of the book of Isaiah describes in beautiful detail this wonderful era. The prophet said, "*. . . and his* [the promised Messiah's] *place of rest will be glorious*" (Isaiah 11:10).

The promise of this glorious time is reassuring and encouraging in a world filled with war, strife, and evil. Each week as the Sabbath is observed, it is a reminder of the unending permanence of God's rest, holiness, and joy.

NUTRITIONAL APPLICATION

Restoration of the Body, Soul, and Spirit

The importance of the balance of the spirit, soul, and body are shown through the three purposes of the Sabbath—rest, holiness and joy. God created a special day that would provide rest (body), holiness (spirit), and joy (soul). This special day—the seventh day—was given a special name, for special purposes, for God's most special creations.

The three Hebrew words most commonly used for *rest* are further evidences of this concept. *Shabath*, from which the word Sabbath is formed, implies ceasing activity, or rest for the body. *Nuwach* infers being settled down with a sense of inner ease, or rest for the soul. *Shaqat* signifies the freedom from external pressures and inner anxiety that only can come through a relationship with God, or rest for the spirit.

In Hebrew thought, all the other days point toward the Sabbath as the pinnacle of the week. How sad that in today's world most people miss the divine significance of the Sabbath!

Restoration of the Body

The rest inherent in the Sabbath is different from the rest provided by the day and night cycle permanently affixed on the fourth day of creation. Unlike the time of sleep when a person does not engage in activity (other than involuntary bodily functions), the rest provided by the Sabbath can be defined better as a time of restoration. Cell phones, e-mails, faxes, pagers, 60 hour work weeks, "extra curricular activities"—we push our bodies beyond the limits of what they were designed to endure then wonder why we feel chronically tired. Stress, a modern epidemic, zaps our strength and hastens the aging process.

God designed our bodies in such a way that the Sabbath innately is a part of our physiological composition. During the moon cycle that occurs from sundown Friday to sundown Saturday (the biblical Sabbath), the heart rate slows and the body naturally goes into a rest mode. Isn't that amazing?

Extra adrenaline is produced when we are in a crisis or sense a dangerous situation. We all have experienced those times when something frightened us and we suddenly experienced an adrenaline rush providing extra strength to avert the danger. Then, when the crisis or danger passed and our adrenaline levels returned to normal, we felt drained of energy.

Unfortunately, most people today live in a constant cycle of stress. Their bodies stay in the crisis mode, rushing to keep schedule demands. The higher adrenaline levels leave the body drained of energy.

Time schedules, as we know them today, were not invented until the nineteenth century. Prior to that, people relied on their inner time—the bodily circadian rhythm mentioned in the beginning chapter. They got up and went to bed with the sun.

The concept of an appointment did not really come into play until 1880 when schedules were created to coincide with the running of the railroad. Until then, time was local. Time on the west coast had no relation to time on the east coast. However, with the creation of the railroad system came the standardization of time as the country was divided into time zones. Then, with the invention of the radio, this concept of standardized time was brought into our homes.

The fifty years between 1880 and 1930 completely overturned our concepts of time. Each decade since then has seen an increase in schedule demands and a decrease in the reliance on the innate sense of inner time. As the gap widens between our internal time clocks and the external time clocks imposed on us by society, the homeostasis of our bodies is destroyed and we experience lives totally out of balance.

Two-thirds of visits to the doctor's office are reported to be stress related. One reason is that the increased flow of adrenaline caused by constant stress will, over a period of time, wreak physical havoc. This chronic flow of increased adrenaline produces some of the following affects on the body:

- High cholesterol
- Narrowing of blood vessels
- Plaque deposits on the walls of the arteries
- Suppression of the immune system

- Production of free radicals in the body.

The Sabbath concept of rest for the body may or may not include extra sleep, but it does include cessation from normal work. It provides an opportunity to step off the merry-go-round, so to speak, and give our bodies a period of time to recover.

Relaxation, a forgotten art in today's society, is a major component in the restoration of the body. It is crucial that we find ways to relax and restore balance to our bodies. The following are some suggestions that might help:

- Sit in a beautiful location outdoors
- Recline in your favorite chair and do nothing
- Listen to relaxing music
- Take a warm bath
- Breathe deeply

However you choose to do it, plan for a time during the Sabbath to rest and restore your body. God certainly knew what He was doing when He showed us—by His example—that the Sabbath was to be a day of rest!

HOLINESS
Restoration of the Spirit

Throughout the Bible we are admonished that the only way to achieve true rest is through God. David says in Psalm 62:1, *"My soul finds rest in God alone."* The Sabbath is a time we can reconnect ourselves with the God who is the source of our rest.

As we rush through life we often find ourselves trying to meet everyone's expectations—except God's. In Galatians 1:10,11 Paul asks, *"Am I trying to win the approval of men, or of God? Or am I trying to please men? If I were still trying to please men, I would not be a servant of Christ."* Our goal should be to please God and not other people.

God never intended for the Sabbath to be laden with rules that would cause it to become a burden. In fact, as was mentioned in the Biblical Application, God gave only one positive and one negative commandment concerning how to keep the Sabbath holy. The positive commandment was that a person should attend a holy convocation, or in today's terminology, a worship service. The negative commandment was that no work should be done on the Sabbath.

Other aspects of how to keep the Sabbath holy were left up to the person to discern. In addition to ceasing work and attending worship, the following are some suggestions for preserving the holiness of the Sabbath (even though these should be daily practices and not just reserved for one day a week):

- **Seek the presence of God.**
  The Puritans taught that there are three aspects of God's presence—essential, cultivated, manifest.
  The **essential presence** of God correlates to His omnipresence. God is everywhere all the time.
  The **cultivated presence** of God concerns those times we sense His presence while seeking Him through private or corporate worship.
  The **manifest presence** involves a supernatural outpouring of His spirit, as during New Testament Pentecost. God has promised in II Chronicles 15:2 that. . . *The Lord is with you when you are with him. If you seek him he will be found by you, but if you forsake him, he will forsake you.*

- **Be quiet.**
  In today's fast paced world, silence is uncomfortable for many people. However, quietude allows us to listen for the *gentle whisper* (I Kings 19:12) of God.
  Being quiet is also an important part of resting. In fact, *quiet* and *rest* are often used interchangeably in Bible passages. Quietness is a meaningful way to rest in God.: . . . *he leads me beside the quiet waters, he restores my soul* (Psalm 23:2).

- **Pray.**
  During times of prayer, we are able to re-focus our priorities. This hectic world easily can lead us to major on the minors. Unimportant things take up valuable time. Prayer reconnects us

to God so that through His spirit we can discern how we should be living the precious gift of life: *May my cry come before you, O Lord; give me understanding according to your word* (Psalm 119:169).

- **Study God's Word.**
  In Hebrew thought, there is a special blessing given to those who study the Torah on the Sabbath. Delighting in the word of God on such a special day helps to replace what the world has taken from us during the week: *I meditate on your precepts and consider your ways. I delight in your decrees; I will not neglect your word* (Psalm 119:15,16).

- **Praise God.**
  Private praise of God is an important theme in the Bible. A natural outpouring of praise will issue forth when time is taken to consider the goodness of God. Praising God for who He is and what He has done also helps us keep our "wish list" in perspective. Gratitude is truly the key to contentment. When we praise God for what we have, we think less about what we do not have: *Be joyful always; pray continually; give thanks in all circumstances, for this is God's will for you in Christ Jesus* (I Thessalonians 5:16-18).

- **Do deeds of kindness as led by the Spirit.**
  In sermons my husband often says, "The cross has a vertical and horizontal dimension, reaching up to God and out to man." As we draw closer to God, He leads us to serve others. Blessing others is yet another way we are blessed on the Sabbath: *The King will reply, "I tell you the truth, whatever you did for one of the least of these brothers of mine, you did for me"* (Matthew 25:40).

The Creation Diet begins and ends with God. The holiness inherent in the Sabbath not only draws us closer to God, it also affects the health of the body and the soul.

JOY
Restoration of the Soul

As I see people rushing through life I have noticed one thing time and again. The expressions on the faces of stressed people do not reflect joy. However, when I see those same people playing in the park with their children or enjoying a meal with family and friends their faces take on a different appearance.

I am reminded of the first year I taught in the high school at a state school for the deaf. It had been a particularly stressful day as I was administering the year-end standardized tests. Trying to explain the directions in sign language and keeping a close watch on the clock for the timed sections was very tiring.

When the tests were completed and passed in, one of my students asked me through signing, "Is your face sick today?" Amused at the phrasing of his question I inquired as to why he thought my face was sick. He replied, "It usually stands there and smiles at us, but today it did not smile much, so I thought it might be sick."

Even though he did not use the "proper" words, this student showed a keen insight. Many people rush through life looking like their faces are sick. How have we allowed our lives to become so stressful that we have lost our joy, and how can we regain it?

The Sabbath provides the answer. The following are some suggestions for discovering or rediscovering the joy God intended for His children to experience.

- **Take the day off.** *You shall not do any work* includes mental as well as physical work.

On the Sabbath, since we are supposed to leave the work of the other six days behind, we also should put the worries of our work behind. It is difficult for humans to grasp the concept of taking time off from regular work to restore the spirit, soul, and body.

In their book Experiencing God, Henry Blackaby and Claude King point out that we are a "doing" people who feel we are only of worth when we are busy doing something. These authors teach that the closer we grow in our relationship to Christ, the less we will feel we must be doing something to be fulfilled and useful.

As it has been said, we are human "beings" not human

"doings." God loves us for who we are, not for what we do. When we grasp the reality of this profound truth, we will find more joy from simply "being" in a relationship with Him than from all the other things we feel compelled to do.

Putting aside work, and the concerns associated with work, will increase our joy and refresh our souls. David expressed it beautifully when he penned, *"I have set the Lord always before me . . . Therefore is my heart glad and my tongue rejoices; my body will also rest secure"* (Psalm 16:8,9).

- **Spend meaningful time with family and friends.**

Throughout its pages the Bible exalts the importance of family and friends. The family was God's first institution. Friends were considered of great value. The Sabbath is a time to reconnect with those we love.

The hectic schedule of a busy workweek often limits the time we have to share with those closest to us. However, the Sabbath is a day designed for corporate worship and meaningful activities with the special people in our lives.

We have many examples in the gospels of Jesus observing the Sabbath with those closest to Him. He regularly attended worship at the synagogue. He walked through grain fields with His friends. He even healed on the Sabbath, bringing joy to others. His example proves that meaningful time with family and friends is an important part of the joy that accompanies the Sabbath.

The concept of joy on the Sabbath is so crucial in Jewish thought that all sadness is banished for that day. If days of fasting fall on the Sabbath they are postponed a day, except Yom Kippur. Since active mourning is forbidden expressly, funerals also are postponed until after the Sabbath.

Yes, rest from work, public and private worship, meaningful time with family and friends, acts of kindness—the Sabbath provides restoration for the spirit, soul and body. The rest, holiness, and joy inherent in the Sabbath help bring balance to our lives even in the midst of a chaotic world.

SPIRITUAL APPLICATION

The Eternal Sabbath

Therefore, since the promise of entering his rest still stands, let us be careful that none of you be found to have fallen short of it. For we also have had the gospel preached to us, just as they did; but the message they heard was of no value to them, because those who heard did not combine it with faith. Now we who have believed enter that rest, just as God has said, "So I declared on oath in my anger, they shall never enter my rest." And yet his work has been finished since the creation of the world. For somewhere he has spoken about the seventh day in these words: "And on the seventh day God rested from all his work." And again in the passage above he says, "They shall never enter my rest." It still remains that some will enter that rest, and those who formerly had the gospel preached to them did not go in, because of their disobedience. Therefore God again set a certain day, calling it Today, when a long time later he spoke through David, as was said before; "Today, if you hear his voice, do not harden your hearts." For if Joshua had given them rest, God would not have spoken later about another day. There remains, then, a Sabbath-rest for the people of God; for anyone who enters God's rest also rests from his own work, just as God did from his. Let us therefore, make every effort to enter that rest, so that no one will fall by following their example of disobedience (Hebrews 4:1-11).

Sabbath-Rest for God's People

The above passage proclaims that one day there will be a Sabbath-rest for God's people. The Sabbath here on earth is actually a foreshadowing of Sabbath-rest in heaven. Again, this rest does not mean inactivity, but rather a state of peace and fulfillment.

The following are some of the characteristics of the eternal Sabbath-rest:

Fulfillment and satisfaction (v. 3,4; 10)

God rested after completing the work of creation. He surveyed His work and declared that *it was very good* (Genesis 1:31). There was a sense of fulfillment and satisfaction within the heart of God.

God did not stop all activity after creation. Certainly He is active every moment of every day working to bring about His ultimate purpose. However, at the conclusion of creation He could cease the labor of creation and enjoy the completion of a job well done.

Someday, for those who enter in the eternal Sabbath-rest God makes available, there will be this same sense of fulfillment and satisfaction. We will complete our work on earth, and enter the heavenly kingdom as we eagerly await to hear the words, *"Well done, good and faithful servant!. . . Come and share your master's happiness!"* (Matthew 25:21)

Deliverance and salvation (v. 5,6)

A strong parallel for Christians is drawn through the Egyptian bondage of the children of Israel, their wilderness wanderings, and their movement toward the promised land of Canaan. In biblical thought, Egypt is representative of the world and its influence. The wilderness wanderings represent the trials and temptations we pass through in life. Canaan represents the land that offers the promise of rest and peace, ultimately heaven.

For those who have chosen to enter into God's eternal Sabbath-rest, we have been delivered from bondage to this world of sin. As we are brought safely through the trials and temptations of daily life conquering the enemies that would beset us, we enter the promised land of rest as free people!

A new and perfect day (v. 7-9)

The children of Israel had kindled the wrath of God when they hardened their hearts at Meribah in the desert and did not believe that God would provide for their needs. Because of this and other acts of disobedience, they were not allowed to enter into Canaan, the promised land.

Almost forty years later when Joshua led the descendants of the children of Israel into the literal Canaan, they experienced a time of temporary rest, or peace. However, soon after they arrived, enemies attacked and they began to fall away from God.

Later, God assured David that there would be a new day of permanent, eternal rest unlike the temporary rest the Israelites had experienced in Canaan. It was promised to all who would *hear his voice* and not *harden your hearts* (v. 7). This new and perfect day would reach its culmination in heaven.

An Urgent Warning

As beautiful and wonderful as the promise of eternal rest is, this passage also is filled with a strong warning that we must be careful not to *be found to have fallen short of it* (Hebrews 4:1). God desires that no one miss the ultimate rest He has provided.

How is it possible to "fall short" of God's eternal rest? This powerful passage clearly explains.

Lack of Faith

First, the gospel of rest has been preached, but some *who heard did not combine it with faith* (v. 2). Every person who hears the gospel has the choice of whether or not to accept it. When our faith accepts God's grace, salvation occurs.

Unbelief

Second, God has *declared on oath* (v. 3) that those who do not believe His promises cannot enter into eternal rest. This is a direct reference to Psalm 95:7-11, which retells the story of how the Israelites hardened their hearts against God in the desert at Massah when they became thirsty. God caused water to flow from a rock at Meribah. However, their lack of belief that God would provide for them after all the miracles they had experienced *tested and tried* God (Psalm 95:9) and evoked His anger.

The greatest example of unbelief is failure to accept God's gracious gift of salvation provided through the cross of Calvary. This unbelief prohibits one from entering in the rest promised to the people of God.

Disobedience

Third, we can fall short of the promise of eternal rest through disobedience. We are told to *make every effort to enter that rest* (v. 11). The Greek word for *effort* is *spoudazzo* meaning "to endeavor, to give all diligence, be zealous, strive eagerly, exert one's self, and make haste."

Nothing in life is more important than our relationship with God. Jesus said in Mark 8:34, *"If anyone would come after me, he must deny himself and take up his cross and follow me."* To disobey that command is to lose the blessed promise of eternal, Sabbath-rest provided for God's people.

In the words of the writer of Hebrews, *"Let us, therefore, make every effort to enter that rest"* (v. 11). Then, at God's appointed time, we can experience the reality of Revelation 14:13: *. . . I heard a voice from heaven say, "Write: Blessed are the dead who die in the Lord from now on." "Yes," says the Spirit, "they will rest from their labor, for their deeds will follow them."*

Dear God of the Sabbath, Creator of the Universe,

Thank you for providing a special day each week that we can rest, focus on You, and engage in meaningful activities with those we love. Thank you for giving us a sign of the importance of this special day by Your example of rest.

Please help us, in some measure, to make the rest, holiness, and joy provided through the Sabbath a part of every day of the week. You are truly the God of the Sabbath, and of each second, moment, hour, day, and week of our lives. We love you!

In Jesus' name I pray, Amen.

MEMORY VERSE FOR CHAPTER SEVEN:
Remember the Sabbath day by keeping it holy (Exodus 20:8).

ASSIGNMENTS FOR CHAPTER SEVEN:

1) **Observe a weekly Sabbath** as a time to focus on God and experience **rest**, **holiness**, and **joy**. Do attend a holy convocation. Do not work.

2) Cultivate **faith, belief**, and **obedience.** (These guard against "falling short" of Sabbath-rest.)

DEVOTIONAL FOR CHAPTER SEVEN

Day One

Scripture Reading: Matthew 26:36-46

Verse of the Day: *Are you still sleeping and resting? Look, the hour is near, and the Son of Man is betrayed into the hands of sinners* (Matthew 26:45).

Today's scripture reading, to me, is one of the saddest in the entire Bible. Jesus observed the Passover meal with His disciples and after the meal, they went to the Garden of Gethsemane. When they arrived there, Jesus took Peter, James, and John apart from the others to support Him and intercede for Him.

He confessed to them that His soul was *overwhelmed with sorrow to the point of death* (Matthew 26:38). Our blessed Savior struggled because He did not want to drink "the cup" that was before Him.

What was "the cup" that so grieved the Son of God? Many people say it was the knowledge of the physical suffering He would experience on the cross. Certainly, that may have been a part of it. Yet I believe it was also the knowledge that He who had never known sin would take on the sins of all people for all time—past, present, and future—and thus would incur the wrath of God. The book of Revelation refers to the cup of God's wrath poured out on evil (Revelation 14:10; 16:19). The holy, innocent, sinless One would in essence experience murder, abortion, hatred, war, violence, genocide, torture, robbery, child molestation, incest, rape, adultery, homosexuality, pornography, robbery, drug abuse, gluttony, lies, deceit, extortion, crime, filthiness, cursing, envy, pride and every imaginable abomination to God. On the cross, Jesus would accept the judgment for our sins and cover them with His precious blood. His sacrificial blood would cleanse and free us from sin's curse forever.

Only love beyond human comprehension would cause Him willingly to accept such atrocities for us. All He asked from Peter, James, and John was that they pray for Him as He agonized over "the cup." He needed them. He needed their prayers on His behalf. He needed them to catch a glimpse of the Father's plan. Three times He returned to them and found them sleeping. Finally, He lamented, *"Look, the hour is near, and the Son of Man is betrayed. . ."* (Matthew 26:45).

Peter, James, and John had missed their golden opportunity. The Savior needed them as never before, and they were too tired to "be there" for Him. They could have helped Him more in that one hour than in the entire three years they followed Him, but they missed their chance. Why? They were simply too tired.

The reality of this passage haunts me. If I do not get adequate rest, I, like Peter, James, and John, am often too tired to do what the Lord is prompting me to do!

Application:
1) List the physical, mental/emotional, and spiritual benefits of rest in your life.
2) Have you ever been too tired to do what you felt the Lord was leading you to do?

PRAY and ask God to show you when and how to best receive His gift of rest.

DEVOTIONAL FOR CHAPTER SEVEN

Day Two

Scripture Reading: Revelation 14:6-13

Verse of the Day: . . . *Blessed are the dead who die in the Lord from now on. "Yes," says the Spirit, "they will rest from their labor, for their deeds will follow them"* (Revelation 14:13).

In cartoons, on Halloween greeting cards, or in scary movies, we are familiar with the sight of a tombstone engraved with the letters "R.I.P." As a child I often wondered how a tombstone was associated with the word "rip." Much later, I learned that it was an abbreviation for "Rest In Peace," which conjures frightening feelings for many people.

However, God's Word teaches that just the opposite should be true. "Rest In Peace" is a promise given to all who *die in the Lord* (v.13). To *die in the Lord* is to have "lived in the Lord." It refers to a person who has received the gift of salvation offered through Jesus' sacrificial death on the cross, and has chosen to follow Him.

Those who die in the Lord are said to be *blessed*, the Greek word *makarios* meaning "supremely blest, fortunate, well off, happy." This is certainly a far cry from the scary "R.I.P." on a lonely tombstone.

Later in Revelation 14:13 we read why those who die in the Lord are well off and happy. They are truly at rest *anapano*, not in the sense of nothingness, but in the sense of "rest and refreshment." They rest **from** the trials, temptations, worries and troubles with which they have labored in this world. They are refreshed **for** the worship, acts of service, and the celestial fun they will experience in heaven.

Many people have the idea that heaven will be somewhat boring, like one eternal church service. It is true that we constantly will be in the presence of God. That in itself will be too glorious to be boring. The earth is beautiful and is filled with many wonderful things to enjoy, but life here is only a tiny preview of what we will experience in heaven.

No eye has seen, no ear has heard, no mind has conceived what God has prepared for those who love him (I Corinthians 2:9). Heaven will be more wonderful than anything we ever have seen, heard, or imagined. No wonder we have to "rest and refresh" to enjoy it!

Another description is in today's scripture passage. For those who choose to follow Satan, there will be *no rest day or night* (Revelation 14:11). Eternal rest or not is determined by whom we choose to worship while on earth.

Application:
1) Describe the kinds of things you would like to do for eternity.
2) Where will you spend eternity? How do you know?

PRAY and thank God for the rest and refreshment He offers believers here and hereafter.

DEVOTIONAL FOR CHAPTER SEVEN

Day Three

Scripture Reading: Psalm 99:1-9

Verse of the Day: *But now that you have been set free from sin and have become slaves to God, the benefit you reap leads to holiness, and the result is eternal life* (Romans 6:22).

Holiness is an interesting word. It is derived from the Hebrew word *qadash* meaning "to be clean ceremonially or morally; consecrate, dedicate, sanctify wholly" and/or the Greek word *hagios* meaning "sacred, physically pure, morally blameless or religious, consecrated." In other words, it means to be "set apart" or "different" from other things. The Sabbath is different from other days, the temple is different from other buildings, and the Christian is different from other men.

However, the most profound aspect of holiness is that God is different from other living beings. God's holiness is His predominant attribute in both the Old and New Testaments. In fact, *holy* is used as a prefix for His name more than any other word.

Scientists tell us that pure, white light is formed when all the colors of the spectrum are combined. Similarly, it can be said that the holiness of God is His essence when all His attributes are combined. God's love, joy, peace, patience, kindness, goodness, faithfulness, gentleness, self-control, righteousness, truth, wisdom, justice, grace, mercy, omnipotence, omniscience, omnipresence, self-existence, and self-sufficiency, when combined, reflect **who** God is and **what** He is—holy.

Paul teaches in Romans 6:22 that once God sets us free from sin we become partakers of His holiness. He dedicates us as different and consecrates us. However, it is our responsibility to live differently from the world, for truly we are set apart for Him.

Recently I met a fine young man and, noticing a beautiful ring on his hand, I questioned him about it. He explained, "This is my promise ring as a commitment to God that I will refrain from having sex until marriage." He is a handsome young man and I am sure there have been and will be many temptations to come his way. Nevertheless, he has vowed to live his life "differently" from the world—"consecrated, physically pure and morally blameless." In other words, he has chosen "holiness."

I have noticed that just as the colors of the spectrum combine to produce pure white light, and the attributes of God combine to form the essence of His holiness, those who are living holy lives also seem to radiate a light. Their eyes sparkle when speaking of their love for Jesus, and they glow when sharing what they have experienced in God's presence. It seems the closer we move to the holiness of God, the more brightly His light shines through us.

Application:

1) Is anyone or anything standing between you and God's holiness?
2) If so, what do you feel God would have you do about it?

PRAY and ask God to help you desire to live a consecrated life of holiness.

DEVOTIONAL FOR CHAPTER SEVEN

Day Four

Scripture Reading: Hebrews 12:1-14

Verse(s) of the Day: *For he chose us in him before the creation of the world to be holy and blameless in his sight. In love he predestined us to be adopted as his sons through Jesus Christ, in accordance with his pleasure and will* (Ephesians 1:4,5).

As a college student, I can remember searching for what seemed to be the illusive "will of God." I read books on the subject and I sought wise counsel from my parents and ministers. My quest to find "God's will" led me to work at our denomination's conference center for the summer. There I attended worship services, talked with missionaries, and spent much time in prayer and Bible study. At that age in life, I thought that "God's will" meant finding the right mate and choosing a career.

Within a few short years, I was married to the person whom I consider to be the most wonderful man in the world and had a fulfilling career as a teacher of the deaf. Those major decisions had been settled, but I found myself still seeking to discover "the will of God." After expecting and not encountering a Damascus Road experience, I realized that "the will of God" is no one thing. "The will of God" is really quite simple. It is that we be adopted as God's children and submit to the authority of our Father. Indeed, it is the culmination of each decision in which we choose to obey God. "A Child of the King" (which was my earthly father's favorite song) is more than a song, it is the will of God!

Today's Verse of the Day emphatically declares this to be true. Before God created the world, He predestined in love for us to be His children and to live holy and blameless lives. The Greek word for *predestine, prooriso*, comes from *pro* meaning "before" and *horizo* meaning "to determine." Therefore, *predestine* literally means "to determine or decree beforehand." Before the world began God decreed that He loved each of us so much He would adopt anyone who would agree to be His child.

The comic strip (and later the movie) "Annie" told the story of a little girl from an orphanage who was adopted by an extremely wealthy man, Daddy Warbucks. The imaginations of millions of people were captured by this "rags to riches" story of a poor girl, adopted by a wealthy, powerful man to live as his child in a beautiful mansion.

We are all "Annies." This world is one huge orphanage, and our wealthy, powerful Heavenly Father desires to adopt us so we can live holy lives as His children and one day live in His home, a beautiful mansion especially prepared for us. This is not a comic strip or a movie. This is "the will of God."

Application:

1) Are you a child of the King? If so, are you living in such a way that others will know who your Father is?
2) If you have not been adopted as a child of God, pray to "legalize" the adoption today. The transaction only can be "signed" with the blood of Jesus!

PRAY and thank God for making it possible to live as "A Child of the King."

DEVOTIONAL FOR CHAPTER SEVEN

Day Five

Scripture Reading: Nehemiah 8:1-18

Verse of the Day: . . . *This day is sacred to our Lord. Do not grieve, for the joy of the Lord is your strength* (Nehemiah 8:10).

"Strength" has become a household word in today's society. "Strength training" exercise equipment, "extra strength" detergents and cleansers, and "maximum strength" pain relievers flood the consumer market. A never-ending search for "strength" occupies the minds and the lives of all ages. However, the Bible clearly gives the formula for strength that is both infallible and eternal—*the joy of the Lord* (Nehemiah 8:10).

After a civil war, the nation of Israel divided into two kingdoms—Israel in the north and Judah in the south. Through various prophets, God warned that those who refused to repent would be taken from their homeland as captives into foreign countries. Continued disobedience led to God's judgment, resulting in Israel's exile into Assyria, and Judah's exile into Babylon.

Today's scripture reading concerns the southern kingdom, Judah. After seventy years of displacement in Babylon, the Jewish captives who desired to return to their beloved homeland were allowed to leave in order to rebuild the temple at Jerusalem.

After rebuilding the temple and the city walls, a scribe named

Ezra held a public reading of God's law, and Nehemiah and the Levites helped explain its meaning.

The people were so moved by what they heard, their remorseful hearts were stirred and they began to weep. The leaders instructed them not to cry but to rejoice, for *the joy of the Lord* would be their strength.

The joy of the Lord—what a wonderful blessing God makes available to us! The Word of God quickens our hearts to mournful repentance, but it also gladdens our hearts by depicting God's mercy and forgiveness. *The joy of the Lord* is founded on a reconciled relationship with God.

Satan tries with all his might to rob us of our joy. He *comes to steal, kill and destroy* (John 10:10) our joy, for he knows that therein is our strength.

One tactic he uses is to get us so focused on our wretchedness as sinners we miss the joy that comes with regeneration. Today's scripture reading is a perfect example, but thankfully we can learn from the people of Judah. Their remorse turned into rejoicing as they observed the Feast of Tabernacles for the first time in many years, affirmed their covenant with God, and denounced their sins: *The sound of rejoicing in Jerusalem could be heard far away* (Nehemiah 12:43). They had regained their joy and strength.

Application:
1) How strong are you in *the joy of the Lord*?
2) What areas of weakness does Satan use against you? What scriptures can combat his personal attacks?

PRAY and ask God to help you focus on His truths rather than Satan's deceptions.

DEVOTIONAL FOR CHAPTER SEVEN

Day Six

Scripture Reading: I Peter 1:3-12

Verse(s) of the Day: *Though you have not seen him, you love him; and even though you do not see him now, you believe in him and are filled with an inexpressible and glorious joy, for you are receiving the goal of your faith, the salvation of your souls* (I Peter 1:8,9).

Life is wonderful! However, life is filled with trials, tribulations, and temptations. We cannot go through life in such a Pollyanna way that we fail to acknowledge the fact that in this world everyone—including Christians—will experience these trials, tribulations, and temptations. We often wonder "why?"

I Peter 1:7 tells us that like gold, we must be *refined* by fire to be proved *genuine. Refined,* in Greek *dokimion,* connotes "to prove; to test; to strengthen." When gold is heated by fire, the impurities float to the surface and can be skimmed off and removed. The product that is left is pure and unadulterated. The same is true of us as we are put through the fires of trials, tribulations, and temptations. They are purposeful. God uses them to make us clean and pure, and to draw us closer to Him.

The result is no less remarkable. Just as pure gold reflects an image, when we are purified and genuine, we reflect Jesus and thus bring *praise, glory, and honor* to Him.

So, how can we know we are genuine? The answer is found in I Peter 1:8,9.

1) Love Jesus, even though we cannot see Him.
2) Believe in Him. The word *believe, pisteuontes,* meaning "to trust," is in the present continuous tense implying "to continue to believe" (even in the midst of trials).
3) Rejoice with the joy that fills our hearts through the Spirit.
4) Keep our eyes focused on the salvation of our souls.

Several years ago I was hiking in the mountains. On the way

down to a beautiful, peaceful waterfall I fell and twisted my knee. I felt I could not make it back up the mountain. As I looked at the vertical trail ahead, it seemed insurmountable. The pain in my knee was intense, but I knew I had to keep climbing. Even though I could not see the summit of the mountain, I knew it was there. So, I chose a rock ahead and stayed focused on climbing to that point. Then I chose another landmark toward which to climb. Finally, I reached the mountaintop and descended the trail to level ground.

In much the same way, we must believe in Jesus although we cannot see Him. Staying focused on what lies ahead helps, even when the way may be difficult and painful.

Application:
1) Are you in the midst of a painful trial, tribulation, or temptation at the present time?
2) What is your main focus? What should it be?

PRAY and thank God for purifying you so you can reflect His image.

DEVOTIONAL FOR CHAPTER SEVEN

Day Seven

Scripture Reading: Zephaniah 3:8-20

Verse of the Day: *The Lord your God is with you, he is mighty to save. He will take great delight in you, he will quiet you with his love, he will rejoice over you with singing* (Zephaniah 3:17).

Rest, holiness, and joy are all represented in Zephaniah 3:17.
Rest—*he will quiet you with his love*
Holiness—*The Lord your God is with you* [within you]
Joy—*he will take great delight in you. . . he will rejoice over you with singing.*

Today's scripture passage comes from a prophetic book in the Bible that pictorially weaves the threat of judgment with the admonition of repentance and the promise of salvation. Zephaniah's exhortation was intended not only for Judah, but also for us and for the entire world: *I have decided to assemble the nations, to gather the kingdoms and to pour out my wrath on them—all my fierce anger. The whole world will be consumed by the fire of my jealous anger* (Zephaniah 3:8) on *the great day of the Lord* (Zephaniah 1:14).

The prophet warned that this time of judgment would be dark and frightening, but the end result would be wonderful. As with most prophetic books of the Bible, Zephaniah presents a two-fold prophecy, a "near fulfillment" and a "future fulfillment."

The "near fulfillment" occurred when Judah was led into captivity—then returned from dispersion a purified and humbled people. The "future fulfillment" will occur when all the nations of the earth praise God in one accord during the Messianic Age.

Nighttime is often a time of fright for young children. As darkness deepens, so do their fears. Nothing quiets the fears of frightened children more than when their parents hold them closely and sing lullabies to them. This special time also blesses the parents as they rejoice over their treasured children.

The great day of the Lord promises to be a frightful day of *darkness and gloom* (Zephaniah 1:15). But, like a parent stealing into the room of a frightened child at night, God also promises to quiet our fears (*he will quiet you with his love*), hold us closely (*The Lord your God is with you*), and, yes, sing to us (*he will rejoice over you with singing*). Rest, holiness, and joy. . . Many times God quiets me with His love, and often I feel Him with me, but I hardly can wait for the time when I hear Him sing!

Application:
1) Has there been a time in your life when something made you so happy that singing was your automatic response? What was it?
2) Are you living in such a way that your obedience would cause God to do the same?

PRAY and thank God for the rest, holiness, and joy that our loving Parent brings.

CHAPTER EIGHT

BIBLICAL APPLICATION

The Creation Diet

As the author of <u>The Creation Diet</u> it is my sincere prayer that this book is a blessing to you. I pray that you have seen a big picture of God as He displayed His glory through the days of creation. I pray also that you have seen a very specific and personal picture of God as He revealed His plan for your well being—spirit, soul, and body.

All the pages of the Bible point to the most important day in all of history. The Old Testament points forward to it through prophecies and foreshadowings, and the New Testament points back to it through historical accounts and doctrinal teachings.

What is this most important day? It is the day when God in the flesh—Jesus the Son—died as the sacrifice for our sins.

Even the days of creation foreshadowed the life, death, burial and resurrection of Jesus. We cannot end the study of the days of creation without delving into these glorious truths!

THE DAYS OF CREATION—FORESHADOWINGS OF JESUS

DAY ONE

LIGHT (HAPPINESS)
Light

As was presented in Chapter One, the *light* spoken into existence on day one was the Hebrew word *owr*, meaning "illumination, including happiness." The light referred to here represents the Shekinah glory of God. Only through a relationship with the Source of light can we experience true happiness.

We are told in scripture that Jesus confirmed Himself to be this light: *When Jesus spoke again to the people, he said, "I am the light of the world. Whoever follows me will never walk in darkness, but will have the light of life"* (John 8:12).

The background of His declaration is especially beautiful. The Feast of Tabernacles, or Sukkot, was one of the three pilgrimages to Jerusalem required of the Hebrews. According to the Mishnah, the Jewish oral tradition, at the end of the first day of the celebration a special ceremony was conducted. The priests and Levites descended to the court of women in the Temple, where four enormous golden candlesticks were set up with four golden bowls placed upon them and four ladders rested against them.

The wicks of these candlesticks were made of worn-out priestly garments. Four young men of priestly descent stood at the top of each ladder holding ten-gallon pitchers of pure oil, which they poured into each bowl at the appropriate time in the ceremony. Amidst festive dances, the playing of instruments, and the singing of praise songs, they lit the oil in the bowls.

The temple radiated so brightly during this lively ceremony, it is said that every courtyard in Jerusalem was lit. Jesus, who was present at this ceremony as recorded in John 8, declared that He is truly *the light of the world*. As beautiful as the temple was, it could in no way compare to Jesus, for *The Son is the radiance of God's glory and the exact representation of his being, sustaining all things by his powerful word. . .* (Hebrews 1:3).

Happiness

There is another remarkable parallel between the light (*owr*) of day one and Jesus' declaration of Himself as *the light of the world* associated with the first day of the Feast of Tabernacles. The light spoken into existence on day one of creation also included the element of happiness, signifying that true happiness can only come from a relationship with God.

The Feast of Tabernacles is noted as being a time of happiness and joy. In fact, it is referred to as "The Season of Our Rejoicing" because it follows the somber observances of Rosh Hashanah, calling for repentance, and Yom Kippur requiring redemption. Through the Feast of Tabernacles, God provided a time for His people to rejoice over their renewed relationship with Him after having passed through the previous seasons of repentance and redemption. After the lighting of the candlesticks on the first day of the Feast of Tabernacles, the Jewish people often sang and danced into the early hours of the morning.

In every sense of the word, Jesus is the true light (happiness) of the world. The statements of the spoken Word of God on day one of creation and the Living Word of God relating to the first day of the Feast of Tabernacles correlate to declare this glorious truth!

SECOND DAY

AIR AND WATER

Air

The first appearance of Jesus to His disciples after the resurrection shows how air created on the second day also points to Jesus. The main purpose of air is to provide living beings with breath. In Hebrew, the word for *breath, neshamah*, also means "spirit." The same is true in Greek. The Greek word for "a current of air; breath," is *pneuma,* which also means "spirit."

John 20:19-23 records that on the night of the resurrection, the disciples (except Judas who had committed suicide and Thomas who was not present) were gathered together behind locked doors, in fear of the same enemies who had crucified their Lord. Jesus appeared to them and assuaged their fears by bringing them a message of peace. He then showed them His hands and side, and they were *overjoyed when they saw the Lord* (John 20:20). Jesus gave them another greeting of peace and commissioned them as His messengers with the words, *"As the Father has sent me, I am sending you"* (John 20:21).

Then Jesus did a remarkable thing. We are told in John 20:22 that He . . . *breathed on them and said, "Receive the Holy Spirit."* Through His divine breath or current of air, the Holy Spirit was imparted to the disciples who were present. This same Spirit would be available to all after Jesus' ascension to heaven. Some Bible scholars suggest that this receiving of the Holy Spirit was like an earnest gift or promise of a fuller indwelling that would come when Jesus was no longer with them.

Breath (current of air) and the Spirit of God are each vital to life. The breath of God gives us life. The breath of Jesus gives us new life. What a beautiful culmination of the purpose of air created on the second day!

Water

The Mishnah describes the ceremony of the water drawing that was conducted on the final day of the Feast of Tabernacles. In the arid land of Israel, rain was considered a blessing from God. The ceremony of the water drawing called upon God to send blessed rain to water the crops.

The ceremony also had a deeper meaning. In many scriptural references water is symbolic of the Holy Spirit. Living water was combined in Jewish thought with the promise of the Messiah and Israel's final redemption as a people, when the Holy Spirit would be poured out upon them. An example of this thought is Isaiah 44:3 which states, *"For I will pour water on the thirsty land, and streams on the dry ground; I will pour out my Spirit on your offspring, and my blessing on your descendants."*

This joyous ceremony began when a specially appointed Levitical priest, surrounded by celebrative worshippers, descended to the pool of Siloam. There he filled a special golden pitcher with water. Then, with the music of flutes and the sound of the shofar trumpet, he and the followers returned to the temple through the Water Gate.

At the southern side of the great altar, he poured the water into a silver basin on the southwest corner of the altar. As the water was poured, the Israelites who had surrounded the altar began chanting the words of Psalm 118:25, *"O Lord, save us; O Lord, grant us success"* and shaking palm branches toward the altar.

Then it happened. At this significant ceremony Jesus made a declaration that would bring hope to every thirsty soul.

> *On the last and greatest day of the Feast, Jesus stood and said in a loud voice, "If anyone is thirsty, let him come to me and drink. Whoever believes in me, as the Scripture has said, streams of living water will flow from within him." By this he meant the Spirit, whom those who believed in him were later to receive. Up to that time the Spirit had not been given, since Jesus had not yet been glorified* (John 7:7-39).

To *drink* the *living water* refers to coming to Jesus in faith. *Streams of living water will flow from within him* conveys the idea of the Holy Spirit indwelling the believer.

Jesus had extended a similar invitation to the woman at the well when He said, *"Everyone who drinks this water will be thirsty again, but whoever drinks the water that I give him will never thirst. Indeed, the water I give him will become in him a spring of water welling up to eternal life"* (John 4:13-14). Now, at the water drawing ceremony during the Feast of Tabernacles, He invited everyone to come and drink of the true *living water*. Through this He announced that He was the promised Messiah who would usher in the time of the outpouring of the Holy Spirit.

Just as the water created on the second day sustains physical life, the *Living Water* of Jesus sustains spiritual life. Even after drinking physical water a person becomes thirsty again. However, after drinking the *Living Water*, an internal spring wells up forever!

THIRD DAY

DRY LAND AND PLANT LIFE

Dry Land

The parallel between the first creation of the third day and the foreshadowing of Jesus can be seen best in His own words to the Pharisees. Matthew 12:40 records that *as Jonah was three days and three nights in the belly of a huge fish, so the Son of Man will be three days and three nights in the heart of the earth.*

Jonah was buried in *the heart of the seas* (Jonah 2:3) for three days and three nights. Likewise, Jesus was in *the heart of the earth* for three days and three nights. (In Hebrew thought a portion of a day counted as a whole day.)

The night before His crucifixion, Jesus prayed in the Garden of Gethsemane with such fervor that *his sweat was like drops of blood falling to the ground* (Luke 22:44). The land He had created received the blood of His agony.

The next day while He was on the cross the ground was soaked with the blood from His wounds. The prophetic Psalm 22 records, *"I am poured out like water, and all my bones are out of joint"* (Psalm 22:14). Once again, the land He had created received His divine blood.

Then the ground accepted His lifeless, blood-stained body as He was buried in a borrowed grave. Paul confirms in I Corinthians 15:3-4 that *for what I received I passed on to you as of first importance: that Christ died for our sins according to the Scriptures, and that he was buried, that he was raised on the third day according to the Scriptures.*

As hard as it is for us to conceive, the very ground God created became Jesus' burial place. The beautiful land He provided for mankind to live was also where He would die. Our daughter, Molly, ends her prayers with, "Lord, help me to **live** as fully for You as You **died** for me." As we walk on this beautiful earth, let us ever be mindful of the fact that this land once held the sacrificed body of God in the flesh—Jesus, our Savior!

Plant Life

Vegetation

The vegetables, seeds, and fruits created on the third day also parallel various descriptions and metaphors associated with Jesus. Throughout the centuries, He has been known lovingly by such names as the Rose of Sharon (Isaiah 35:1; Song of Songs 2:1).

However, two of the most poignant parallels associated with plant life and the life of Jesus come from the seed category (the Bread of Life) and the fruit category (the Vine).

Seeds

In John's gospel we read,

> *Then Jesus declared, "I am the bread of life. He who comes to me will never go hungry, and he who believes in me will never be thirsty (John 6:35). For I have come down from heaven not to do my will but to do the will of him who sent me. And this is the will of him who sent me, that I shall lose none of all that he has given me, but raise them up at the last day. For my Father's will is that everyone who looks to the Son and believes in him shall have eternal life, and I will raise him up at the last day" (John 6:38-40).*

We read that many of the Jewish hearers began to grumble wondering how He could say that He *came from heaven* (John 6:41). In response Jesus answered,

> *"I am the bread that comes down from heaven. Your forefathers ate the manna in the desert, yet they died. But here is the bread that comes down from heaven, which a man may eat and not die. I am the living bread that came down from heaven. If anyone eats of this bread, he will live forever. This bread is my flesh, which I will give for the life of the world"* (John 6:48-51).

As we have repeatedly seen in The Creation Diet, God used physical things and events in the Hebrew Scriptures to foreshadow the spiritual truths of the New Testament. The *Bread of Life*, also known as *Living Bread*, is no exception.

In Exodus 16:4 God told Moses, "*. . . I will rain down bread from heaven for you. The people will go out each day and gather enough for that day. In this way I will test them and see whether they will follow my instructions.*" It appears that since in this verse God said, "*I will rain down*," the children of Israel expected to find particles of God on earth.

The Hebrew word for "manna" is *mawn* meaning, "a whatness" (so called from the question about it): *When the Israelites saw it they said to each other, "What is it?" For they did not know what it was. Moses said to them, "It is the bread the Lord has given you to eat"* (Exodus 16:15).

The etymology of the word *manna* is rich and beautiful. In his book entitled Manna, Karl D. Coke explains that the word *manna* is comprised of the two Hebrew words *mahn* and *hu*. *Mahn* is from an unused Hebrew root word meaning, "divide or allot, part or portion, it is a portion." *Hu* in Hebrew is the personal pronoun equivalent to the English word, "he." In essence, the Israelites expected to see "a portion of Him." It is little wonder that when they saw bread they questioned, "What is it?"

Praise God, one day He did "rain down" in a manger in Bethlehem (which means "House of Bread") as had been foreshadowed in the Desert of Sin thousands of years previously! All who will accept His provision indeed have "a portion of Him" living inside of them. This is the *Living Bread*, and the *Father's will is that everyone who looks to the Son and believes in him shall have eternal life. . .* (John 6:40).

It is important to note that the provision of manna was given one day at a time, each morning, except for the double provision on the day before the Sabbath (Exodus 16:5). God's plan is that we depend upon the *Living Bread* daily for our sustenance!

We are reminded of this each time we partake of Holy Communion, often referred to as the Lord's Supper. The element of the broken bread is symbolic of the *Living Bread* whose body was broken for all who will receive.

Fruits

John's gospel records Jesus' words,

I am the true vine, and my Father is the gardener. He cuts off every branch in me that bears no fruit, while every branch that does bear fruit he prunes so that it will be even more fruitful. You are already clean because of the word I have spoken to you. Remain in me, and I will remain in you. No branch can bear fruit by itself; it must remain in the vine. Neither can you bear fruit unless you remain in me. I am the vine; you are the branches. If a man remains in me and I in him, he will bear much fruit; apart from me you can do nothing. If anyone does not remain in me, he is like a branch that is thrown into the fire and burned. If you remain in me and my words remain in you, ask whatever you wish, and it will be given you. This is to my Father's glory, that you bear much fruit, showing yourselves to be my disciples" (John 15:1-8).

This passage confirms that the Father is the Gardener, Jesus is the Vine, and believers are the branches. The Gardener plants and tends the Vine. In turn, the Vine is the life of the fruit. Apart from the Vine there is no life and no fruit.

As the branches, believers either bear *no fruit* (John 15:2), *fruit* (John 15:2), *more fruit* (John 15:2), or *much fruit* (John 15:5,8).

What is the "fruit" that is referred to here? The answer is found throughout passages in the New Testament. The fruit is *righteousness* (Philippians 1:11); *good works* of righteousness (Colossians 1:10); *fruit of the Spirit* or Godly character (Galatians 5:22-23); and new believers (Romans 1:13).

The secret of how much fruit a believer bears is simple. It depends upon how closely the branch stays attached to the Vine. Apart from Jesus we can do nothing. It is only when we *remain* (John 15:5) in Him that we are able to bear fruit. His very essence flows through us and the natural outcome of this nourishment is *fruit*.

The end result is that the Gardener will be glorified. Bringing glory to the Father was Jesus' main objective while on earth. For those who remain in Him, the same will be true.

FOURTH DAY

SUN, MOON AND STARS

The purposes of heavenly bodies created on the fourth day foreshadow the ministry of Jesus. In Genesis 1:14 God said, *"Let there be lights in the expanse of the sky to separate the day from the night, and let them serve as signs to mark seasons and days and years."* The sun, moon and stars were created with four main purposes—to separate the day from the night, signs, seasons, days and years. We see that the purposes are glimpses of the Messiah.

Separate Day from Night
John's gospel records some of the most poignant words in the Bible concerning the separation of the light of day and the darkness of night.

> *In him was life, and that life was the light of men* (John 1:4). *The light shines in the darkness, but the darkness has not understood it* (John 1:5). *This is the verdict: Light has come into the world, but men loved darkness instead of light because their deeds were evil. Everyone who does evil hates the light, and will not come into the light for fear that his deeds will be exposed. But whoever lives by the truth comes into the light, so that it may be seen plainly that what he had done has been done through God* (John 3:19-21).

These passages show clearly that there is a choice between darkness and light. Jesus is the light. Those who choose to live in relationship with Him become children of light.

Therefore Paul could say to the believers at Thessalonica, *"You are all sons of the light and sons of the day. We do not belong to the night or to the darkness*" (I Thessalonians 5:5). Just as the sun, moon and stars separated day from night physically, Jesus does the same for believers spiritually.

Signs
The Christmas story beautifully paints the picture of how Jesus in the flesh was a sign that redemption had come into the world.

> *And there were shepherds living out in the fields nearby, keeping watch over their flocks at night. An angel of the Lord appeared to them, and the glory of the Lord shone around them, and they were terrified. But the angel said to them, "Do not be afraid. I bring you good news of great joy that will be for all people. Today in the town of David a Savior has been born to you; he is Christ the Lord. This will be a sign to you: you will find a baby wrapped in cloths and lying in a manger"* (Luke 2:8-12).

The shepherds were told that the Baby in the manger was a sign that the promised Messiah, the Christ, had been born. As we consider that Jesus Himself was the long awaited sign, with the angels we can exclaim, *"Glory to God in the highest, and on earth peace to men on whom his favor rests"* (Luke 2:14).

Seasons
The Hebrew word for seasons, *mowed* means "an appointment (a fixed time or season); festival." The life of Jesus clearly fulfills each of these meanings of the word "seasons."

An appointment; a fixed time; or season
No matter what the appointment, the fixed time, the season, Jesus has been, is now, and will be there. He transcends time. In Revelation 1:8, our Lord declares that He is the One "... *who is and who was, and who is to come, the Almighty*".

Seasons come and seasons go, yet He remains forever: *Do not be afraid. I am the First and the Last. I am the Living One; I was dead, and behold I am alive forever and ever! And I hold the keys of death and Hades* (Revelation 1:17-18).

Festival, An Assembly; Feast

Jesus proclaimed in Matthew 5:17, *"Do not think that I have come to abolish the Law or the Prophets; I have not come to abolish them but to fulfill them."* As an observant Jewish man, Jesus kept the law as set forth in the Torah. We read of Him observing the various festivals as recorded in Leviticus 23.

There were three pilgrimages the Jewish people were to make to observe festivals in Jerusalem. These were the feasts of Passover (Deuteronomy 16:5), Pentecost and Tabernacles. Scripture shows us Jesus' adherence to these mandates.

Luke's gospel tells us that annually Jesus and his parents went to Jerusalem for the Feast of the Passover: *When he was twelve years old, they went up to the Feast, according to the custom* (Luke 2:41-42).

John records an early account in the ministry of Jesus: *Now while he was in Jerusalem at Passover Feast, many people saw the miraculous signs he was doing and believed in his name* (John 2:23).

All four gospels record that Jesus was in Jerusalem observing Passover when He was arrested and killed (Matthew 26:17-18; Mark 14:12-16; Luke 22:7-13; John 13:1).

In addition to Passover, it is verified through scripture that Jesus observed other festivals as well. John 7:1-39 attests to the fact that Jesus observed the Feast of Tabernacles in Jerusalem. He even kept Hanukkah, also called the Feast of Lights and/or the Feast of Dedication, which was added during the 400 years between the Old and New Testaments: *Then came the Feast of Dedication at Jerusalem. It was winter, and Jesus was in the temple area walking in Solomon's Colonnade* (John 10:22).

In conclusion, the major events of Jesus' life followed the calendar of Jewish Festivals. He died on Passover, was in the grave on Unleavened Bread, and rose on First Fruits. The church, the Bride of Christ, was birthed on Pentecost (Acts 2:1).

Many scholars believe that the Feast of Trumpets foreshadows the time Jesus' Bride will join Him, in what is known as "the rapture"

(I Thessalonians 4:13-18). Also it is believed that the great tribulation (Revelation 6-19) corresponds to Yom Kippur, and His second coming is equated with the Feast of Tabernacles (Revelation 20:1-6).

In addition, there is a growing body of belief that Jesus, the Light of the World, was conceived of the Holy Spirit on Hanukkah, the Feast of Lights, and that He was born during the Feast of Tabernacles. When John's gospel records that *the Word became flesh and made his dwelling among us . . .* (John 1:14), the Greek word *dwelling* is *akenoo* meaning "to tent or encamp or specifically to reside (as God did in the Tabernacle of old, a symbol of protection and communion.)" In other words, *the Word became flesh and* "tabernacled" *among us.*

As His own words declare, Jesus did come to fulfill and not to abolish or destroy the Law. Through the Festivals of Leviticus 23 a picture is drawn which foreshadows the most significant events in His life and, indeed, in the history of the world.

Days and Years

As *days and years* are indicative of the passing of time, scripture records Jesus' words, ". . . *I am the Alpha and the Omega, the Beginning and the End. . .*" (Revelation 21:6).

He pre-existed time: *In the beginning was the Word, and the Word was with God and the Word was God* (John 1:1).

His advent split history. His birth is the indicator that marks time, B. C. "before Christ" and A. D. "after Christ" (from the Latin phrase Anno Domini, meaning "in the year of the Lord.")

He is *the Beginning and the End.* He is *the First and the Last* (Revelation 1:17). He is. . . *alive for ever and ever! . . .* (Revelation 1:18).

FIFTH DAY

FISH AND FOWL

As with the other elements of the creation narrative, the living beings called forth into existence on the fifth day are further correlations of the life and death of Jesus. The fish and fowl point to important aspects about Him.

Fish

Although scripture records, *And God said, "Let the water teem with living creatures . . ."* (Genesis 1:20), God said that humans would have *rule over the fish of the sea . . .*(Genesis 1:26). Since the word *fish* is specially used, we will look at how that relates to our Savior.

The primary Greek word for *fish* in the New Testament is *ichthus*. A significant fact is associated with this word. If an acrostic is compiled from the first letters of each of the words in the phrase, "Jesus Christ, Son of God, Savior," the word *ichthus* is formed. Because of this, the Greek word for *fish* was important to the early church. Believers would secretly draw the sign of the fish to let others know of their allegiance to Jesus.

The Greek letters of *fish* became a sacred acrostic that is still used today by believers. God would give the same mandate to believers today that He spoke to the fish on the fifth day of creation, " *. . . Be fruitful and increase in numbers . . .* " (Genesis 1:22).

Fowl

An often over-looked truth profoundly is recorded in John's gospel. It concerns an encounter with John, the forerunner, who is referred to also as John the Baptist due to his mandate for the baptism of repentance.

> *Then John gave this testimony: "I saw the Spirit come down from heaven as a dove and remain on him. I would not have known him, except that the one who sent me to baptize with water told me, 'The man on whom you see the Spirit come down and remain is he who will baptize with the Holy Spirit.' I have seen and I testify that this is the Son of God"* (John 1:32-34).

The dove was considered a sacred bird to the Jewish people. Even though it was a symbol of peace and purity, it was more often identified with the Spirit of God.

Prior to Christ, the Spirit did not abide continually with men, but came upon them for special purposes and at special occasions. Old Testament individuals were said to have experienced a special visitation of the Spirit.

Those who experienced this anointing of the Holy Spirit in the Hebrew Scriptures are as follows:

Joseph (Genesis 41:38), Moses (Numbers 11:17), Joshua (Numbers 27:18), Othniel (Judges 3:10), Gideon (Judges 6:34), Jephthah (Judges 11:29), three times upon Samson (Judges 14:6; Judges 14:19, Judges 15:14-15), twice upon Saul (I Samuel 10:10; I Samuel 11:6), David (I Samuel 16:13), Elijah (I Kings 18:12), Elisha (II Kings 2:15), Ezekiel (Ezekiel 2:2), Daniel (Daniel 4:9), Micah (Micah 3:8), Azariah the prophet (II Chronicles 15:1), Zechariah the high priest (II Chronicles 24:20), the seventy elders of Israel (Numbers 11:25), the children of Israel in the desert (Nehemiah 9:20).

God revealed to John that when the Holy Spirit came upon a Man in the form of a dove and remained, he would recognize that Man as the promised Messiah. A significant truth is that the dove, representing the Holy Spirit, remained on Jesus. It did not just descend and then return to heaven. In essence, it represented the Spirit of God Himself descending upon Jesus, filling Him with power and authority and remaining with Him. Symbolically, the dove became a part of Him.

The good news is that on this side of the cross the same it true for those who accept Jesus Christ as Savior and Lord. They become children of God. Paul wrote in Romans 8:9-10, *"You however, are controlled not by the sinful nature but by the Spirit, if the Spirit of God lives in you. And if anyone does not have the Spirit of Christ, he does not belong to Christ. But if Christ is in you, your body is dead because of sin, yet your spirit is alive because of righteousness."*

What a glorious thought for Christians to realize! The dove has lighted upon us, and it remains. Like Jesus, we are empowered to live life to the fullest. Then, we can look forward to the day we too will hear God say, *"This is my Son* [child], *whom I love; with him* [or her] *I am well pleased."*

SIXTH DAY

LIVESTOCK (Cattle KJV), CREATURES THAT MOVE ALONG THE GROUND (Creeping thing KJV), WILD ANIMALS (Beast of the earth KJV) AND MAN

Livestock (Cattle KJV)

The most significant livestock in Hebrew history were sheep, specifically lambs used for sacrificial purposes as well as for food. The ewe is the female lamb and the male lamb is called a ram.

When John the forerunner saw Jesus he exclaimed ". . . *Look, the Lamb of God, who takes away the sin of the world!*" (John 1:29) John stated that this *Lamb of God* was the One of whom he had prophesied.

Years later another John, who had been one of Jesus' disciples, was given a vision of heaven while he was exiled on the island of Patmos. In his vision he saw the Lamb of God being worshipped by the angels, living creatures, and elders around the throne: *In a loud voice they sang: "Worthy is the Lamb, who was slain, to receive power and wealth and wisdom and strength and honor and glory and praise!"* (Revelation 5:12)

What characteristics of a lamb correlate with the *Lamb of God*? First of all, sheep quickly learn to recognize the voice of the shepherd and follow him. Jesus Himself said,

> *The man who enters by the gate is the shepherd of his sheep. The watchman opens the gate for him, and the sheep listen to his voice. He calls his own sheep by name and leads them out. When he has brought out all his own, he goes on ahead of them, and his sheep follow him because they know his voice. But they will never follow a stranger; in fact, they will run away from him because they do not recognize a stranger's voice* (John 10:2-5).

Like a lamb, Jesus heeded and obeyed the voice of His Father, the Shepherd. He said, *"And the Father who sent me has himself testified concerning me"* . . . (John 5:37). *"For I have come down from heaven not to do my will but to do the will of him who sent me"* (John 6:38).

Jesus' whole life, ministry, and sacrificial death were in obedience to the voice of His Father. He clearly knew the Father's will for His life: *For my Father's will is that everyone who looks to the Son and believes in him shall have eternal life, and I will raise him up at the last da*y (John 6:40).

Not only did Jesus recognize the Father's will for His life, he submitted to that will. The night before the crucifixion He prayed, *"Father, if you are willing, take this cup from me; yet not my will, but yours be done"* (Luke 22:42).

The result of His obedience is that *everyone who looks to the Son and believes in him* (John 6:40) can be made righteous: *For just as through the disobedience of the one man* [Adam] *the many were made sinners, so also through the obedience of the one man* [Jesus] *the many will be made righteous* (Romans 5:19).

A second characteristic of a lamb is that it can be led to its death without a struggle. In fact, it has been reported that many times when the Priests cut the throat of the sacrificial lambs according to the Kosher method of slaughter, the lambs licked the hands of the very ones who were killing them.

Similarly, our Lord laid down His life with a spirit of submission and humility: *And being found in appearance as a man, he humbled himself and became obedient to death—even death on a cross!* (Philippians 2:8) Jesus said of His life, *"No one takes it from me, but I lay it down of my own accord"* (John 10:18).

The Hebrew word for *livestock, behemah,* comes from an unused root that probably means "to be mute." What a beautiful foreshadowing of how Jesus faced His death! We are told in I Peter 2:23 that *When they hurled their insults at him, he did not retaliate; when he suffered, he made no threats.* This was an allusion to a Messianic prophecy in Isaiah 53:7 that *He was oppressed and afflicted, yet he did not open his mouth; he was led like a lamb to the slaughter, and as a sheep before her shearers is silent, so he did not open his mouth.*

Jesus as the sacrificial Lamb for all time willingly died so that we might live. When we realize the eternal significance of this, we like the heavenly beings should shout, *"Worthy is the Lamb!"*

Creatures that move along the ground (creeping thing KJV)
As I was considering how the life of Jesus was foreshadowed in the days of creation, I could not imagine how *creatures that move along the ground* (or a *creeping thing*) could relate to our Savior. While researching, I found some information that not only amazed me but showed me anew how miraculous the Word of God is.

Probably when we think of *creatures that move along the ground*, snakes are the first things that come to mind. After the fall, the serpent, or snake, was told by God, *"Because you have done this, cursed are you above all the livestock and all the wild animals! You will crawl on your belly and you will eat dust all the days of your life"* (Genesis 3:14).

Another time in scripture snakes were associated with a curse. Because the children of Israel complained against Moses and against God while they were in the wilderness, God sent poisonous serpents among them and the people began to die from the snakebites.

They repented and called out to God for deliverance: *God then told Moses, "Make a snake and put it up on a pole; any one who is bitten can look on it and live"* (Numbers 21:8).

Moses did as God instructed: *So Moses made a bronze snake and put it up on a pole. Then when anyone was bitten by a snake and looked at the bronze snake, he lived* (Numbers 21:9). "Bronze" and "brass" are interchangeable in the Bible.

Just before His death, Jesus compared this account from the Torah with His impending death. He said, *"Just as Moses lifted up the snake in the desert, so the Son of Man must be lifted up, that everyone who believes in him may have eternal life"* (John 3:14).

The snake had been the cause of death, yet a serpent made of brass *lifted up* would be the means of deliverance. Even so, Jesus became sin for us. When *lifted up* on the cross of Calvary, He also became the means of deliverance: *He himself bore our sins in his body on the tree, so that we might die to sins and live for righteousness; by his wounds you have been healed* (I Peter 2:24).

Throughout scripture brass, or bronze, is associated with God's judgment of sin. Some examples are as follows:

- The brass altar was used in the temple for the sin offerings (Exodus 38:30).
- After the fall of mankind, God told the serpent, *"And I will put enmity between you and the woman* [Eve], *and between your offspring and hers; he will crush your head and you will strike his heel"* (Genesis 3:15).
- In John's vision of heaven, his description of Jesus is that *"His feet were like bronze flowing in a furnace. . ."* (Revelation 1:15).

The brass snake was fastened to a pole and lifted up. Our Lord and Savior was fastened to a pole and lifted up.

The Hebrew word for "snake" is *nachash* and the word for "bronze" or "brass" is *nachashet*. The Hebrew alphabet characters are thought to be pictures of things. The last letter of the Hebrew alphabet, *tav* (ת) is believed to be a cross. When the *tav*, or cross, is added to the word for "snake" the word changes and becomes "brass."

What a beautiful insight the Hebrew language gives us. When Jesus was *lifted up* on the cross, He took on Himself God's judgment on sin. Hallelujah, what a Savior!

Wild animals (Beast of the earth KJV)

Jesus, the humble Lamb of God, is associated also with the king of the jungle, a lion. Throughout scripture He is called the Lion of Judah. What characteristics about His life lead to such a comparison?

First, Judah refers to His earthly ancestry. Even though Jesus was conceived of the Holy Spirit, He was a part of an earthly family. King David was from the tribe of Judah (Matthew 1:3-6). Jesus *belonged to the house and line of David* (Luke 2:4). This affirms that Jesus was from the tribe of Judah.

Secondly, in passages where Jesus is called the Lion of Judah, His ministry corresponds with the traits normally thought of as belonging to a lion. It is believed that the tribal symbol of Judah was a picture of a lion.

The lion is considered the king of the jungle for several reasons. One is that he is the king of predatory beasts. He is able to destroy his enemies. Our Lion of the Tribe of Judah has done precisely that for us.

Satan tries to be the "king of the jungle." I Peter 5:8 warns, "*Be self-controlled and alert. Your enemy the devil prowls around like a roaring lion looking for someone to devour. . .*" However, *the reason the Son of God appeared was to destroy the devil's work* (I John 3:8). What a comforting assurance!

In John's vision, he witnessed the fact that no one in heaven was worthy to break the seals and open the scroll, believed by many scholars to be the deed to the earth. The opening of the scroll would usher in the events leading to a time of great tribulation and ultimately the restoration of all things. John was broken-hearted that no one was worthy to open the scroll.

> *I wept and wept because no one was found who was worthy to open the scroll or look inside. Then one of the elders said to me, "Do not weep! See the Lion of the tribe of Judah, the Root of David, has triumphed. He is able to open the scroll and its seven seals"* (Revelation 5:4-5).

The Lion of Judah, the *King of kings and Lord of lords* (Revelation 19:16) triumphed over the enemy. He won the victory!

How did He do it? John explains in Revelation 5:6, when he said, "*Then I saw a Lamb, looking as if it had been slain, standing in the center of the throne. . .*" The Lamb *that was slain from the creation of the world* (Revelation 13:8) destroyed the enemy by giving His own life's blood. The forces of evil are powerless against the blood of Jesus. No wonder our Lamb boldly proclaimed, "*I was dead, and behold I am alive for ever and ever! And I hold the keys of death and Hades*" (Revelation 1:18).

Yes, the Lion of Judah has triumphed over sin and death. Therefore, . . . *Death has been swallowed up in victory* (I Corinthians 15:54). The Lion of Judah reigns!

Man

The correlation between Jesus and God's final creation is also one of the most humbling. The love that caused the Son of God to become the Son of Man is beyond human comprehension. I bow in amazement as I consider the incarnation, when *the Word became flesh and made his dwelling among us* . . . (John 1:15).

Man was God's most special creation. God *crowned him with glory and honor and put everything under his feet* (Hebrews 2:7-8). In fact, man was created only *a little lower than the angels* (Hebrews 2:7).

When man sinned, his natural body became *perishable, dishonorable and weak* (I Corinthians 15:42-43). His heart became *deceitful above all things* (Jeremiah 17:9).

God provided a way to renew mankind: *For the life of a creature is in the blood, and I have given it to you to make atonement for yourselves on the altar; it is the blood that makes atonement for one's life* (Leviticus 17:11). He allowed an animal to be presented as a substitution for sacrifice on behalf of the sinner. However, even this was pointing ahead to the time that God Himself would come to earth as the final sacrifice for all who would accept His unprecedented gift.

Since blood was necessary for atonement, He became flesh and blood so that He could give His life's blood to save mankind: *Since the children have flesh and blood, he too shared in their humanity so that by his death he might destroy him who holds the power of death—that is the devil—and free those who all their lives were held in slavery by their fear of death* (Hebrews 2:14).

We can rest assured that *when this priest had offered for all time one sacrifice for sins, he sat down at the right hand of God* (Hebrews 10:12). The priests were not allowed to sit down until their work was completed. Jesus, having completed the work of salvation on the cross, sat down at the right hand of the Father. *It is finished* (John 19:30) now and forevermore.

"Son of Man" was the title by which Jesus referred to Himself more than any other. Paul clearly showed the humility of our Savior when he penned the words,

"Your attitude should be the same as that of Christ Jesus: Who, being in very nature God, did not consider equality with God something to be grasped, but made himself nothing, taking the very nature of a

servant, being made in human likeness. And being found in appearance as a man, he humbled himself and became obedient to death—even death on a cross!" (Philippians 2:5-8)

My heart is broken as I think that the Son of God became the Son of Man for me. Then my heart rejoices as I realize that,

Therefore God exalted him to the highest place and gave him the name that is above every name, that at the name of Jesus every knee should bow, in heaven and on earth and under the earth, and every tongue confess that Jesus Christ is Lord, to the glory of God the Father (Philippians 2:9-11).

SEVENTH DAY

SABBATH REST

As we come to the final day in the creation narrative, we see that this day also paints a beautiful picture of Jesus, the Messiah. In Him we find the Sabbath rest that God modeled when . . . *God blessed the seventh day and made it holy, because on it he rested from all the work of creating that he had done* (Genesis 2:3).

Rested in this verse is the Hebrew word *shabath* from which the word "Sabbath" is derived. It means, "to repose, for example, to desist from exertion."

Jesus offers this rest in Matthew 11:28-30: *Come to me, all you who are weary and burdened, and I will give you rest. Take my yoke upon you and learn from me, for I am gentle and humble in heart, and you will find rest for your souls. For my yoke is easy and my burden is light.*

The first *rest* Jesus offers in this passage is the Greek word *anapauo* meaning, "to give rest, quiet, recreate, refresh." It indicates the rest that comes from salvation. The unbeliever, weary from bondage to sin and heavy-laden with sin's consequences, is told simply to *"Come unto me." Come* is the Greek word *deute* and is an imperative verb meaning, "come hither; come follow."

Jesus tells the sinner to come and follow Him. The result is that their personal weariness from the heavy burden of sin will be lifted, and He will give them rest, quiet, recreation and refreshment.

The second *rest* offered by Jesus is *anapausis* and it means, "rest; inward tranquility while one performs necessary labor." Why is this rest necessary?

Jesus says to *take my yoke upon you and learn from me*. The yoke is a powerful symbol in the Bible. Literally, it refers to a cattle yoke that binds animals to a plow, and often to each other. Symbolically it speaks of "servitude or an obligation."

Once we accept the salvation Christ offers, we come under His authority to learn from Him. The more we learn from Him, and the more we emulate what we have learned, the more like Him we become. Through this learning He provides a lifelong pursuit that gives meaning to each day of our existence on earth.

Jesus says that His *yoke is easy* and His *burden is light*. The Greek work for *easy* is *chrestos* implying "well-fitted." Cattle yokes that do not fit well rub against the shoulders of the animals and injure their skin. Jesus knows which yoke is best for us, and in His love He places a well-fitted yoke upon us.

In first century Judaism, the people were familiar with the symbolism of the yoke. The "yoke of Torah" was the obligation to keep the Law. However, the Pharisees had added man-made interpretations of that law that weighed down the people. Jesus assured that His yoke was different. It was well-fitted. It did not weigh one down with man-made interpretations of the Law.

Jesus' *burden* is the Greek word *phortion* and it figuratively means "a task or service." The tasks He gives are light in comparison to the burden of what the world requires of us. Our Savior does not release us from the responsibilities associated with being a follower of His. Instead, through the indwelling of the Holy Spirit, He provides the best way for us to carry them: *This is love for God to obey his commands. And his commands are not burdensome, for everyone born of God overcomes the world. This is the victory that has overcome the world, even our faith* (I John 5:3-4).

What is the result of coming to Jesus and taking His yoke? *You will find rest for your souls.* "Inward tranquility while one performs necessary labor" . . . the necessary labor of submitting to the authority of a holy, loving Savior. What more could anyone ask?

Rest, Holiness and Joy

The three elements inherent in the final day of creation are exemplified by the promises of our Savior. Rest, holiness and joy are vital lessons to *learn from* Him as we take His yoke upon us.

Rest

From Matthew 11:28-30 we see that coming to Jesus and putting on His yoke offers a rest that the world can never give. As Jesus said, it is a *rest for your souls*. This "rest of the soul" restores and refreshes our minds and emotions.

Guilt is replaced with a feeling of purification. *If we confess our sins, he is faithful and just and will forgive us our sins and purify us from all unrighteousness* (I John 1:9).

Anxiety is replaced with peace. *Peace I leave with you; my peace I give you. I do not give to you as the world gives. Do not let your hearts be troubled and do not be afraid* (John 14:27).

Fear is replaced with love. *There is no fear in love. But perfect love drives out fear . . .* (I John 4:18).

Doubt is replaced with hope. *Christ in you, the hope of glory* (Colossians 1:27).

Holiness

Taking on the yoke of Jesus and entering into His blessed rest leads to holiness which is not available by any other means: *But just as he who called you is holy, so be holy in all you do; for it is written, "Be holy, because I am holy"* (I Peter 1:15). Any attempts to be holy apart from a relationship with Jesus will only fail. Holy God became man so that man might partake in His holiness. The more we *learn from Him* the more we will have an understanding of how to lead holy lives.

Joy

We are told in scripture that . . . *the joy of the Lord is your strength* (Nehemiah 8:10). Experiencing the presence of the Lord results in joy. When Jesus instructed us to *learn of me*, He understood that obeying His commandments would bring us into His presence and resting there would make our joy complete:. . . *Now remain in my love. If you obey my commands, you will remain in my love, just as I have obeyed my Father's commands and remain in his love. I have told you this so that my joy may be in you and that your joy may be complete* (John 15:9-11).

Rest, holiness, joy . . . easy yoke and light burden! Are you weary and burdened? Come unto Him and receive blessed rest.

NUTRITIONAL APPLICATION

The assignments given at the end of each chapter form the basis of The Creation Diet. God reveals through creation how to live step-by-step balanced in spirit, soul and body. When we adhere to these principles we can develop our relationship with God, attain a healthy mind and emotions, and achieve physical vitality.

Before presenting a summary of The Creation Diet I would like to share some insights which can help us to adhere to its principles. Keeping these suggestions in mind can mean the difference between health and wholeness or disease and distress.

1) Schedule a specific time to spend with God.
If we do not develop a planned time to meet with God, we tend to postpone our fellowship with Him. It seems the visible things dominate our lives yet an encounter with the invisible God is the most important thing we can do to maintain balance in life.

Many people say the reason they do not spend intimate time with God is that they really do not know how. If you find that true in your own life, perhaps the following suggestions will help:

The following acrostic is as an example of how to spend time with God:

Prepare your heart.
Spend some time thanking God for His blessings in your life. Read and meditate upon Bible passages that seem to bring you closer to God. Listen to music that prepares your heart for worship.

Repent

Ask God to reveal to you anything that keeps you from an awareness of His presence. Acknowledge to God that you recognize it as sin and ask Him to help you remove it from your life.

Adore

Spend time adoring God for who He is. Reflect upon His attributes. (Holiness, goodness, love, understanding, patience, wisdom, power, mercy and grace are but a few of His attributes.) This is a time to worship Him. Singing to God is a wonderful way to adore Him.

Yield to His will.

Present your requests for yourself and others to Him and trust that He will do what is best in each situation.

Bible study can come either at this time or at a later time in the day. The purpose of this "quiet time" is to commune with God.

2) Accentuate the positive.

On any given day we are exposed to more negatives than positives. To maintain balanced lives, it is vital that we learn to dwell on the positives. Most problems in life arise either from misperception or miscommunication. We must remember that believers have *the mind of Christ* (I Corinthians 2:14). Therefore, with His mind we can perceive the good in even seemingly bad situations.

Reading positive and affirming books and listening to uplifting music help accentuate the positive. Also, associating with people who have a healthy outlook on life will help us focus on the right things.

We need to give ourselves permission to celebrate our strengths and not feel that we are egotistical for doing so. Since psychologists report that 90% of what we tell ourselves about ourselves is negative, self-affirmations throughout the day can help change that statistic.

As stated in Chapter One, the first two minutes of the day set the tone for the remainder of the day. Disciplining ourselves to dwell on uplifting thoughts the first thing upon waking each morning prepares us for a more positive day.

3) Surround yourself with wholesome foods.

We need to "spring clean" our kitchens and rid them of unwholesome foods that tempt us. In their places, we need to re-stock our kitchens with wholesome foods. The following are some essentials for healthy eating:

Fresh vegetables (or quick frozen)
Whole-grain breads and pastas (gluten free is best for most people)
Brown rice
High fiber cereals with a minimal amount of sugar (around 5 grams)
Fresh, raw nuts (Almonds are wonderful.)
Organic nut butters
Dried beans
Olive oil for cooking
Sea salt (rather than regular processed salt)
Honey
Stevia
Herbs and spices to flavor foods
Fresh fruits (or quick frozen)
Fish from fresh water sources
Eggs from free-range poultry
Free-range poultry naturally processed
Meat raised and processed without chemicals
Organic Certified raw dairy products

Because fresh vegetable juices contain live enzymes and a host of other nutrients, it would be worth the investment to buy a good juicer. These are suggestions to help turn our kitchens into places where we prepare "meals that heal."

THE CREATION DIET

The Creation Diet is more a way of life than a set plan or program. Although it is an overall plan for a balanced body, each person is unique and should consider the foods and the serving sizes that are best for them.

What Counts as a Serving?

According to <u>The Creation Diet</u> the following are the suggested amounts that constitute a serving:

WATER
8 ounces

VEGETABLES
1 cup of raw leafy vegetables
½ cup of chopped raw vegetables
½ cup of cooked vegetables
¾ cup of vegetable juice

SEEDS
⅓ to ½ cup of seeds
1 slice of bread
1 ounce of ready-to-eat cereal
½ cup of cooked cereal, rice, or pasta
½ cup of cooked dry beans

OILS
1 Tablespoon

FRUITS
1 medium piece of fresh fruit
½ cup of berries
½ cup of chopped fruit
¾ cup of fruit juice (diluted with water)

DAIRY
1 cup of yogurt (or cottage cheese)
1½ ounces of natural cheese
1 Tablespoon of butter
8 ounces of milk

MEAT
2-3 ounces of cooked lean fish, poultry, or meat
1 egg

Fiber Content

Books and charts are available that show the nutritional content of different foods. The following amounts are a good estimate when considering which foods offer the highest amount of fiber per serving:

Cooked dried beans have approximately 7 grams
Seeds and nuts have approximately 3-5 grams (almonds have 6 grams)
Rice has 2 grams
Pasta has 2 grams
Vegetables have 2 grams
Fruits have 2 grams

Alkaline and Acidic Foods

After food is digested and the nutrients removed, an end product called "ash" is left in the tissues for some time. Ash is either alkaline or acidic, depending upon the foods eaten.

Foods that produce an alkaline ash (above pH 7.0) in the body are called "base-forming" foods, and foods that produce acid ash (below pH 7.0) are called "acid-forming" foods. The body functions best in a slightly alkaline environment. (7.2-7.365 pH)

Although the research is still in process and lists and charts vary, the following is a good summary of alkaline and acidic foods.

Foods that leave an **alkaline ash** in the body are as follows:
* **Vegetables (most)**
* **Some unprocessed seeds (flax, pumpkin, squash, sunflower, and sprouted seeds)**
* **Almonds and chestnuts**
* **Fruits (other than cranberries and blueberries)**
* **Raw whey and raw cattle (goat and cow) milk**

Foods that leave an **acid ash** in the body are as follows:
* **Animal proteins**
* **Processed dairy products**
* **Most nuts (with the exception of almonds and chestnuts)**

- **Whole grains (except millet and quinoa)**
- **Legumes**
- **Vegetable oils**

The following substances leave no ash (because they supply no nutrients to be metabolized), but they have an **acidifying effect** on the body:

- **Alcohol**
- **Tobacco**
- **Drugs/medications**
- **Syrups**
- **Saturated fats**
- **Hydrogenated oils**
- **Sugars (processed)**
- **Artificial sweeteners**
- **Processed grains**
- **Table salt**
- **Drinks containing caffeine**

THE CREATION DIET

The Creation Diet is comprised of the principles that are presented in each chapter related to the days of creation. A summary of the overall program is as follows:

LESSONS FROM DAY ONE (*Genesis 1:1-5*) LIGHT AND HAPPINESS

1) **Focus on God** first thing in the morning, last thing at night, and throughout the day. Establish a time each day for prayer and Bible study and worship.

2) **Think happy thoughts.** Make a conscious effort to replace negative thoughts with positive ones—thought by thought.

LESSONS FROM THE SECOND DAY (*Genesis 1:6-8*) **AIR AND WATER**

3) Perform at least **10 deep breathing exercises** a day. **Deep breathing**, preferably **fresh air**, throughout the day will help oxygenate the blood.

4) **Water** should be consumed throughout the day, with a goal of at least **8 ounces per 20 pounds of body weight.** (Divide your body weight by 20 to determine the number of 8 ounce glasses of water you should drink daily.)

LESSONS FROM THE THIRD DAY (*Genesis 1:9-13*) **PLANT FOODS**

5) **Increase** the amount of **alkaline-ash** foods you consume by choosing **5-7 servings of vegetables (primarily non-starchy or low glycemic).**

6) Also, include **2-3 servings of fruits** in your diet daily.

Although not substantiated through Scripture, modern research shows that fruits eaten alone pass quickly through the stomach (in twenty to thirty minutes). However, when combined with other foods, their presence in the stomach causes digestive juices to begin to spoil animal protein foods and ferment carbohydrates. A good motto for consumption of fruits is "eat them alone or leave them alone."

7) **Decrease** the amount of food you eat from the **acid-ash group**. Since most vegetables from the seed category — **some seeds, most nuts, whole grains and legumes** — leave an acid ash but are high in fiber, carefully choose **3-5 servings** from this category daily. Choose high-fiber, low-acid foods.

Remember: Your goal is to choose a large percentage (many nutritionists say 75%) of your foods from the

alkaline-ash group.

8) **Consume 1-2 Tablespoons** daily of **cold-pressed vegetable oils** as good sources of essential fatty acids.

9) **Include raw plant foods daily**, preferably with each meal.

LESSONS FROM THE FOURTH DAY (*Genesis 1:14-19*) **SUN, MOON, STARS**

10) Spend time each day in the **fresh air and sunshine.** Gradually build up to **30 minutes per day** outdoors when the sun's rays are not direct.

11) Determine the amount of **sleep** your body requires, approximately **1/3 of the day (8 hours).** If you presently are not getting enough sleep, begin the process of adjusting your bedtime by going to bed fifteen minutes earlier progressively until you are getting adequate rest.

12) **Develop your relationship with God** and participate in **meaningful religious observances.**

13) Choose servings of **vegetables** (5-7), **seeds** (3-5), and **fruit** (2-3) from a **variety of colors.** Take advantage of the seasonal foods that are available.

14) Determine to make **life-style choices** that will ensure **health and fulfillment** as you age. Remember that God created you with a purpose in mind, even before you were in your mother's womb. **Seek God's guidance daily**, finding your intended purpose as you progress through the seasons of life.

LESSONS FROM THE FIFTH DAY (*Genesis 1:20-23*) **FISH AND FOWL**

15) **Seek healthful sources** of fish and poultry.

16) Limit intake to **1 to 1 ½ servings (3-4 oz.) daily** of "clean" **fish** or "clean" **fowl**. This amounts to a serving approximately the size of a deck of cards.

17) Consumption of **fresh eggs** from "free range" chickens should be limited to **one egg daily,** including those in cooked foods.

LESSONS FROM THE SIXTH DAY (*Genesis 1:24-31*) LAND ANIMALS AND MAN

18) Limit animal products. **Eat red meat of livestock (*cattle*) sparingly.** Also, find unadulterated sources for the meat.

19) **One serving of plain yogurt, kefir, butter, or natural cheese, cottage cheese,** or **buttermilk** (all of which are similar to the biblical *curds*) may be consumed **daily.** The most healthful sources are unpasturized and unhomogenized. Consumption of liquid goat's milk and cow's milk should be limited, and should come from organic, certified, raw sources. An alternative to animal milk is vegetable milk. Good sources include rice, almond, and natural non-hybrid soy milk.

20) Commit to **moderate exercise** at least **five days per week.**

LESSONS FROM THE SEVENTH DAY (*Genesis 2:1-3*) THE SABBATH

21) **Observe a weekly Sabbath** as a time to focus on God and experience **rest, holiness,** and **joy.** Do attend a holy convocation. Do not work.

22) Cultivate **faith, belief**, and **obedience to God.**

In Hebrew, the number 22 is representative of light. Isn't that amazing?

TO LOSE WEIGHT

The Creation Diet is an overall plan for health rather than a weight-reduction program. However, temporarily eliminating the elements of the **Seed Category** (seeds, nuts, whole grains, and legumes) except for the healthful essential fatty acid oils will aid weight loss. After two weeks of eliminating these foods, reintroduce them in lesser amounts than the suggested serving size one at a time as desired.

In addition, choose vegetables that do not convert to sugar easily. High glycemic vegetables such as white potatoes, corn, and carrots should be eliminated or at least limited while trying to lose weight.

ONE DAY AT A TIME

Making lifestyle changes may seem overwhelming at first. However, once again, God has shown us a beautiful pattern of how to bring balance into our lives.

He created the world one day at a time. Likewise, we can re-create our personal worlds one day at a time.

When we choose to obey God day-by-day, over a period of time those days accumulate and we will find that we have positively affected our futures!

SPIRITUAL APPLICATION

As we come to the end of The Creation Diet, I pray this will be the beginning in the following ways:

For those of you who have never accepted the gift of God's love through Jesus Christ and His atoning sacrifice on the cross of Calvary, I pray this will be the beginning of your relationship with Him.

For those of you who are believers, but who have strayed from His paths, I pray this will be the beginning of a renewed fellowship with Him.

For those of you who need to make lifestyle changes to protect and preserve your body—His temple—I pray this will be the beginning of a new way of healthy living.

More than anything else with the writing of <u>The Creation Diet</u> I have desired to reveal the truth of God's Word—the Bible— and to show God's remarkable plan for each of us. Every element of the creation narrative points to God's majesty. Every element of the Bible points to God's love through Jesus Christ.

PLAN OF SALVATION
Relationship

God created us in His image so that we could live in close relationship with Him and constantly experience His presence. Adam and Eve, the first man and woman, were created perfectly in spirit, soul, and body. They had an intimate relationship with God and were able to experience the full joy of His presence.

However, they chose to disobey God and eat of the tree of the knowledge of good and evil (Genesis 3:6). Until then, all they had ever known was good, but at the moment of disobedience, evil became part of them also. Like a mutant gene, that same evil, also known as unrighteousness, has been passed on to every person in each succeeding generation. The Bible says, *"There is no one righteous, not even one"*. . . (Romans 3:10).

Righteous God cannot live in relationship with unrighteous man. Our unrighteousness separates us from holy God and prevents us from experiencing the joy of His presence. God's justice demands that unrighteousness must be punished and eliminated in order for Him to live in relationship with us. However, there is nothing we could ever do on our own to make ourselves righteous before God.

So, in an unprecedented act of unconditional love, God came to earth in human form through Jesus Christ and took the punishment for our unrighteousness. On the cross, all of the evil that separated us from God was placed on Him and He bore it in our place: *God made him who had no sin to be sin for us, so that in him we might become the righteousness of God* (II Corinthians 5:21).

Jesus gave His own blood to pay the price that the penalty of our sin required. His atoning death is a gift given freely to all who will receive it: *For the wages of sin is death, but the gift of God is eternal life in Christ Jesus our Lord* (Romans 6:23).

God desires to live in relationship with us so much that He will share His righteousness with us. He will change us to be like Him if we choose to let Him. . . *put on the new self, created to be like God in true righteousness and holiness* (Ephesians 4:24).

How does this change occur? It happens when we are *born again* (John 3:7). Just as we were born physically on a certain date, in order to *enter the kingdom of heaven* (John 3:5) we must also be born spiritually. It is a supernatural miracle initiated and completed by God Himself. When we respond by faith to what God has done on the cross of Calvary, we are *born again*.

If you have never entered into relationship with God through spiritual birth, please do not delay any longer . . . *now is the time of God's favor, now is the day of salvation* (I Corinthians 6:2).

Admit your unrighteousness. *For all have sinned and fall short of the glory of God* (Romans 3:23).
Believe that Jesus' death on the cross makes you righteous before God. *This righteousness from God comes through faith in Jesus Christ to all who believe. . .* (Romans 3:22).
Confess that you accept God's gift of salvation and dedicate your life to Him. *For God so loved the world that he gave his one and only son, that whoever believes in him shall not perish but have eternal life* (John 3:16).
Depend upon the Holy Spirit to guide your decisions. *For the kingdom of God is not a matter of eating and drinking, but of righteousness, peace and joy in the Holy Spirit* (Romans 14:17).

Fellowship

Fellowship with God is another term for our closeness to Him. Once we have been *born again*, we are in relationship with Him. However, our fellowship with Him depends upon the choices we make.

It is much like a marriage. Once a man and woman marry, they are in the relationship of marriage. However, their closeness to each other depends upon the level of their expression of love for each other. Once we have entered into relationship with God through His atoning death on the cross, our purpose in life is to develop our fellowship with Him. As in a marriage, our fellowship is dependent upon the level of our expression of love for God. Obedience is the way we express our love for God. When we choose to obey Him by rejecting evil and developing characteristics that are like Him our fellowship is one of joy.

It's All About the Cross

Being raised as an Egyptian, Moses had been told of many different pagan "gods." However, He encountered **the** God at the burning bush and was commissioned to deliver the Israelites from bondage in Egypt. He asked a significant question of God: *"Suppose I go to the Israelites and say to them, 'The God of your fathers has sent me to you,' and they ask me, 'What is his name?' Then what shall I tell them?"* (Exodus 3:13)

God's answer to that question was, *". . . You shall say to the children of Israel, I AM has sent me to you"* (Exodus 3:14). In Hebrew, which originally had no vowels, *I AM* is יהוה (*Yahweh*).

The Hebrew alphabet letters represent pictures of different objects. The letters can either be the actual object or the function of the object. Since Hebrew reads from right to left, in looking at the name of God we see that the first letter (י) represents a hand. The second letter (ה) represents, among other things, a window. Therefore, it can also represent "look," or "behold" since a window is used for looking. The third letter (ו) represents a nail or a hook.

Even the name of God given to Moses at the burning bush foreshadows the cross. As the picutre of the letters are joined, *I AM*, means "Hand-Behold-Nail-Behold."

In addition, there was a specific reason the angel told Mary in Matthew 1:21, *". . . You are to give him the name Jesus, because he will save his people from their sins."* Jesus' name in Hebrew is ישוע (*Yeshua*). In Jesus' name the message becomes more specific. Again the first letter (י) represents a hand. The second letter (ש) when used alone stands for *Shaddai*, meaning "Almighty God." The third letter (ו) represents a nail or a hook. The fourth letter (ע) represents an eye. (It is believed that originally it was shaped more like an eye.) Therefore, it can represent the function of the eye that is to "look" or "behold."

As the pictures of the letters of Jesus' name are joined they declare "Hand-Almighty God-Nail-Behold." The prophecy of the angel was fulfilled for truly He saved *his people from their sins* when the hand of Almighty God was nailed to the cross of Calvary. Hallelujah, what a Savior!

Where is Your Heart?

The first recorded question in the Bible is the one God asked Adam after he had sinned: *But the Lord God called to the man, "Where are you?"* (Genesis 3:9)

God asked Adam a rhetorical question. As has been shown many times throughout The Creation Diet, God is omniscient. He is all knowing. He knew exactly where Adam was.

A more literal rendering of the Hebrew is "Where is your heart?" God knew where Adam was physically, but He wanted Adam to face the question of his spiritual condition. God would ask the same of each of us today.

In Hebrew there is a basic shape that is the foundation of two different letters. If the dot is placed on the right side (שׁ) it is the *shin*, the "*sh*" sound. (We do not have an equivalent letter in English.) Whenever the *sh* is used alone it represents *Shaddai*, "Almighty God."

If the dot is placed on the left side of the shape (שׂ) it is the *sin*, the "*s*" sound. Words such as "Satan" and "sin" begin with that letter.

Blaise Paschal, the French mathematician and philosopher wrote that each person is born with a God-shaped void. A cross-section of the human heart reveals that it is literally the same shape of the two letters. In a real since, we make the choice of where the dot goes, depending upon whom we choose to serve.

The Human Heart
An echocardiogram of my precious husband's heart

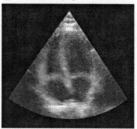

As <u>The Creation Diet</u> concludes I leave each reader with the same question God asked of the first man: "Where is your heart?"

FOR MORE INFORMATION
For more information on <u>The Creation Diet</u> and related products or the author, Joy Clary Brown, visit the website at www.the creationdiet.com

Selected Bibliography

Some of the sources used in the writing of this book are as follows:

Biblical Resources:

Unless otherwise stated the New International Version was used for scripture references and Abingdon's Strong's Exhaustive Concordance of the Bible was used for the Hebrew and Greek words.

Hebrew Greek Key Word Study Bible, New International Version, AMG, 1996.

The Visualized Bible, King James Version, Wheaton, Illinois, Tyndale House Publishers, Inc., 1985.

Strong, James, The Exhaustive Concordance of the Bible, Nashville, Tennessee, Abingdon, 1890.

The Pulpit Commentary, Grand Rapids Michigan, Wm. B. Eerdmans Publishing Company, 1958.

The Preacher's Outline and Sermon Bible, New Testament, New International Version, Chattanooga, Tennessee, 1998.

Other Resources:

Appleton, Nancy, Ph.D., Lick the Sugar Habit, Garden City Park, New York, Avery Publishing Group, 1996.

Baldinger, Kathleen O'Bannon and Richards, Larry, Ph. D., Health & Nutrition God's Word for the Biblically-Inept, Lancaster, Pennsylvania, Starburst Publishers, 1999.

Baldinger, Kathleen, O'Bannon, The World's Oldest Health Plan, Lancaster, Pennsylvania, Starburst Publishers, 1994.

Barnhart, Clarence, The World Book Dictionary, United States, Doubleday & Company, Inc., 1967.

Booker, Richard, The Miracle of the Scarlet Thread, Shippensburg, Pennsylvania, Destiny Image Publishers, 1981.

Brand, Paul, Dr. and Yancey, Philip, Fearfully and Wonderfully Made, Grand Rapids, Michigan, Zondervan Publishing House, 1980.

Bullinger, E. W., The Witness of the Stars, Grand Rapids, Michigan, Kregel Publications, reprint of the 1893 edition, 2000.

Childers, Greer, Be a Loser, United States of America, Times Books, 1998.

Cloutier, Marissa, M.S., R.D. and Adamson, Eve, The Mediterranean Diet, New York, New York, Harpertorch, 2001.

Cooper, Kenneth H., M.D., Antioxidant Revolution, Nashville, Tennessee, Thomas Nelson, Inc., 1994.

Darden, Ellington, Ph. D., A Flat Stomach ASAP, United States of America, Pocket Books, 1998.

Davis, Karen, Ph.D., <u>Prisoned Chickens Poisoned Eggs</u>, Summertown, Tennessee, Book Publishing Company, 1996.

Dement, William C., M.D., Ph.D. and Vaughan, Christopher, <u>The Promise of Sleep</u>, New York, New York, Delacorte Press, 1999.

Diamond, Harvey, <u>Fit For Life A New Beginning</u>, New York, New York, Kessington Books, 2000.

Fuchs, Daniel, <u>Israel's Holy Days in Type and Prophecy</u>, Neptune, New Jersey, Liozeaux Brothers, 1985.

Graci, Sam, <u>The Power of Superfoods</u>, Scarborough, Ontario, Prentice Hall Canada Inc., 1999.

Jeffrey, Grant R., <u>The Signature of God</u>, Nashville, Tennessee, Word Publishing, 1998.

Kasdan, Barney, <u>God's Appointed Customs</u>, Baltimore, Maryland, Lederer Books, 1996.

Keller, Phillip, <u>A Shepherd Looks At Psalm 23</u>, Grand Rapids, Michigan, Zondervan Publishing House, 1970.

Kennedy, Peter with Colby, Brenda and Espinosa, Lorraine, <u>From Generation to Generation</u>, Uhrichsville, Ohio, Barbour Publishing, Inc., 1998.

Klingman, Patrick, <u>Finding Rest When the Work Is Never Done</u>, United States of America, Victor Cook Communications, 2000.

Kuzma, Jan W. and Cecil Murphey, <u>Live 10 Healthy Years Longer</u>, Nashville, Tennessee, Word Publishing, 2000.

Levitt, Zola, <u>The Seven Feasts of Israel</u>, Zola Levitt, 1979.

Luton, L. Grant, <u>In His Own Words</u>, Akron, Ohio, Beth Tikkun Publishing, 1999.

McFarland, Judy Lindberg, <u>Aging Without Growing Old</u>, Lake Mary, Florida, 2003.

Malkmus, George H., Dr. with Michael Dye, <u>God's Way to Ultimate Health</u>, Shelby, North Carolina, Hallelujah Acres Publishing, 1995.

Meinz, David L., M.S. R.D. F.A.D.A., C.S.P, <u>Eating by the Book</u>, Virginia Beach, Virginia, Gilbert Press, 1999.

Omartian, Stormie, <u>Greater Health God's Way</u>, Eugene, Oregon, Harvest House Publishers, 1996.

Robbins, John, <u>Diet for a New America</u>, Tiburon, California, H. J. Kramer, 1987.

Rowe, John W. M.D. and Kahn, Robert L., Ph. D., <u>Successful Aging</u>, New York, New York, Dell Publishing, 1999.

Rubin, Jordan, S. N. M. D., Ph. D., <u>The Maker's Diet</u>, Lake Mary, Florida, Siloam, 2004.

Russell, Rex, M.D., <u>What the Bible Says About Healthy Eating</u>, Ventura, California, Regal Books, 1996.

Smolenshky, Michael and Lambery, Lynne, <u>The Body Clock Guide to Better Health</u>, New York, New York, Henry Holt & Company, 2000.

Tessler, Gordon S., Ph. D., <u>Breaking the Fat Barrier</u>, Raleigh, North Carolina, The Genesis Way, Inc., 1993.

Zimmerman, Martha, <u>Celebrate the Feasts</u>, Minneapolis, Minnesota, Bethany House Publishers, 1981.